The SAGES Manual

D1524908

The SAGES Manual

A Practical Guide to Bariatric Surgery

Ninh T. Nguyen, MD

Associate Professor of Surgery, Chief, Division of Gastrointestinal
and Bariatric Surgery, University of California, Irvine Medical Center,
Orange, CA, USA

Editor-in-chief

Eric J. DeMaria, MD

Professor and Vice Chairman, Network General Surgery,
Director, Bariatric and EndoSurgery,
Duke University, Durham, NC, USA

Sayeed Ikramuddin, MD

Associate Professor of Surgery, Co-Director,
Minimally Invasive Surgery, Director, Gastrointestinal Surgery,
Katherine and Robert Goodale Chair in Minimally Invasive Surgery,
University of Minnesota, Minneapolis, MN, USA

Matthew M. Hutter, MD, MPH

Director, Codman Center of Clinical Effectiveness in Surgery,
Department of Surgery, Massachusetts General Hospital,
Boston, MA, USA

Editors

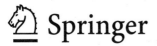 Springer

Ninh T. Nguyen, MD
Associate Professor of Surgery
Chief, Division of Gastrointestinal
   and Bariatric Surgery
University of California
Irvine Medical Center
Orange, CA
USA

Eric J. DeMaria, MD
Professor and Vice Chairman
Network General Surgery
Director, Bariatric and EndoSurgery
Duke University, Durham, NC
USA

Sayeed Ikramuddin, MD
Associate Professor of Surgery
Co-Director
Minimally Invasive Surgery
Director, Gastrointestinal Surgery
Katherine and Robert Goodale
   Chair in Minimally Invasive Surgery
University of Minnesota
Minneapolis, MN
USA

Matthew M, Hutter, MD, MPH
Director, Codman Center of Clinical
   Effectiveness in Surgery
Department of Surgery
Massachusetts General Hospital
Boston, MA
USA

ISBN: 978-0-387-69170-1   e-ISBN: 978-0-387-69171-8

Library of Congress Control Number: 2008936875

Preface

The field of bariatric surgery has grown at an exponential rate over the past decade. The number of bariatric operations has increased from less than 10,000 operations in 1998 to nearly 200,000 operations in 2008. Bariatric surgery has become an integral part of gastrointestinal surgery and is now an important part of education for surgical residents and fellows in minimally invasive surgery. Educational initiatives in bariatric surgery take many different forms and currently many textbooks on the topic of bariatric surgery are commercially available. However, there is a need for a quick-reference manual that provides up-to-date, easy access to information about this new and complex surgical specialty.

The SAGES Manual: A Practical Guide to Bariatric Surgery began as a project developed within the SAGES Bariatric Liaison group. The name of the book previews its primary purpose, as it is meant to provide practical information within a small pocket-sized book that can serve as a portable resource anywhere, including the ward and clinic. This manual provides a concise, practical guide to promote high-quality, safe care for patients undergoing weight loss surgery. It is intended to be used by any members of the multidisciplinary team, including surgeons, surgeons-in-training, medical physicians, medical students, nurses, nurse practitioners, physician's assistants, nutritionists, and psychologists.

We would like to thank members of the SAGES Bariatric Liaison group who have contributed to the manual, the SAGES leadership whose support and encouragement were critical for its development, and Springer for helping to make this project a reality. Our goal is that knowledge gained from using this manual will help to promote safe and effective care for patients undergoing bariatric surgery.

Ninh T. Nguyen, MD
Eric J. DeMaria, MD
Matthew M. Hutter, MD, MPH
Sayeed Ikramuddin, MD

Contents

II. Techniques

III. Outcomes

IV. Complications

V. Guidelines and Accreditation in Bariatric Surgery

Contributors

Jamie D. Adair, MD
Department of Surgery, St. Joseph Mercy Oakland Hospital,
Bloomfield Hills, MI

Helmuth T. Billy, MD
Director of Bariatric Surgery, St. John's Regional Medical Center,
Ventura Advanced Surgical Associates, Ventura, CA

Robin P. Blackstone, MD, FACS
Clinical Associate Professor of Surgery, University of Arizona School
of Medicine-Phoenix, Medical Director, Scottsdale Bariatric Center,
Scottsdale, AZ

Stacy A. Brethauer, MD
Staff Surgeon, Bariatric and Metabolic Institute, Cleveland Clinic,
Cleveland, OH

Bipan Chand, MD
Director, Surgical Endoscopy, Bariatric and Metabolic Institute,
Cleveland Clinic, Cleveland, OH

Peter F. Crookes, MD
Associate Professor of Surgery, University of Southern California,
Department of Surgery, University Hospital, Los Angeles, CA

Eric J. DeMaria, MD
Professor and Vice Chairman, Network General Surgery, Director,
Bariatric and EndoSurgery, Duke University, Durham, NC

Bradley T. Ewing, PhD
Rawls Endowed Professor of Operations Management, Texas Tech
University, Rawls College of Business, Lubbock, TX

Edward L. Felix, MD
Advanced Bariatric Center, Assistant Clinical Professor,
UCSF-Fresno, Director of Bariatric Surgery, Clovis Community
Medical Center, Fresno, CA

Eldo E. Frezza, MD, MBA, FACS
Professor, Texas Tech University Health Sciences Center, Chief
of General Surgery, University Medical Center, Lubbock, TX

Michel Gagner, MD, FACS, FRCSC
Chairman, Department of Surgery, Mount Sinai Medical Center, Miami
Beach, FL

Rolf Gordhamer, PhD
Psychologist and Consultant, Texas Tech University, Lubbock, TX

Giselle G. Hamad, MD, FACS
Assistant Professor of Surgery, University of Pittsburgh School
of Medicine, Department of Surgery, Magee-Women's Hospital
of UPMC, Pittsburgh, PA

Daniel M. Herron, MD
Associate Professor of Surgery, Mount Sinai School of Medicine, Chief,
Section of Bariatric Surgery, Mount Sinai Medical Center, New York, NY

Marcelo W. Hinojosa, MD
Resident Physician, Department of Surgery, University of California,
Irvine Medical Center, Orange, CA

Matthew M. Hutter, MD, MPH
Director, Codman Center for Clinical Effectiveness in Surgery,
Department of Surgery, Massachusetts General Hospital, Boston, MA

Sayeed Ikramuddin, MD
Associate Professor of Surgery, Co-Director, Minimally Invasive
Surgery, Director, Gastrointestinal Surgery, Katherine and Robert
Goodale Chair in Minimally Invasive Surgery, University of Minnesota,
Minneapolis, MN

Thomas H. Inge, MD, PhD
Associate Professor of Pediatrics and Surgery, University of Cincinnati,
Department of Pediatric General & Thoracic Surgery, Cincinnati
Children's Hospital Medical Center, Cincinnati, OH

Daniel B. Jones, MD
Associate Professor, Chief, Section of Minimally Invasive Surgery,
Harvard Medical School, Director, Bariatric Program, Beth Israel
Deaconess Medical Center, Boston, MA

Orit Kaidar-Person, MD
The Bariatric and Metabolic Institute, Cleveland Clinic Florida, Weston, FL

Marina Kurian, MD
Assistant Professor of Surgery, New York University School of Medicine,
Department of Surgery, New York University Medical Center,
New York, NY

Andrew B. Lederman, MD, FACS
Medical Director of Bariatric Surgery, Berkshire Medical Center,
Assistant Professor of Surgery, University of Massachusetts Medical
School, Pittsfield, MA

Xingxiang Li, MD
The Bariatric and Metabolic Institute, Cleveland Clinic Florida,
Weston, FL, Department of Minimally Invasive Surgery, Shanghai
Changhai Hospital, Shanghai, China

Troy A. Markel, MD
General Surgery Resident, Indiana University School of Medicine,
Indianapolis, IN

Samer G. Mattar, MD, FRCS, FACS
Associate Professor of Surgery, Department of Surgery, Indiana University School of Medicine, Clarian North Medical Center, Indianapolis, IN

Ross L. McMahon, MD, FRCSC, FACS
Medical Director, Department of Bariatric Surgery, Swedish Medical
Center, Seattle, WA

Marc P. Michalsky, MD, FACS, FAAP
Assistant Professor of Clinical Surgery, Ohio State University,
Department of Pediatric Surgery, Nationwide Children's Hospital,
Columbus, OH

Dean J. Mikami, MD
Assistant Professor of Surgery, The Ohio State University, Department
of Minimally Invasive Surgery, Ohio State University Hospital,
Columbus, OH

Go Miyano, MD
Fellow, Department of Pediatric General & Thoracic Surgery,
Cincinnati Children's Hospital, Cincinnati, OH

John M. Morton, MD, MPH, FACS
Director of Bariatric Surgery, Stanford University Medical Center,
Stanford, CA

Murali N. Naidu, MD
Associate Physician, The Permanente Medical Group, Antioch, CA

Bradley J. Needleman, MD, FACS
Assistant Professor of Surgery, The Ohio State University, Director, Bariatric
Surgery, The Ohio State University Medical Center, Columbus, OH

Ninh T. Nguyen, MD
Associate Professor of Surgery, Division of Gastrointestinal and Bariatric
Surgery, University of California, Irvine Medical Center, Orange, CA

Manish Parikh, MD
Clinical Fellow in Laparoscopic and Bariatric Surgery, Weill Medical
College of Cornell University, Department of Surgery, New York
Presbyterian Hospital, New York, NY

Alexander Perez, MD
Minimally Invasive Surgery Fellow, Duke University Medical Center,
Durham, NC

Mark A. Pleatman, MD
Attending Physician, St. Joseph Mercy Oakland, Pontiac, MI

Alfons Pomp, MD, FRCSC, FACS
Leon C. Hirsch Professor of Surgery, Chief, Section of Laparoscopic
and Bariatric Surgery, Weill Medical College of Cornell University,
New York Presbyterian Hospital, New York, NY

Janey S.A. Pratt, MD, FACS
Instructor of Surgery, Harvard University School of Medicine,
Department of Surgery, Massachusetts General Hospital, Boston, MA

David A. Provost, MD
Associate Professor, Division of Gastrointestinal Endocrine Surgery,
University of Texas Southwestern Medical Center, Dallas, TX

Raul J. Rosenthal, MD, FACS
Director, Bariatric Institute, Department of General and Minimally
Invasive Surgery, Cleveland Clinic Florida, Weston, FL

Philip R. Schauer, MD
Professor of Surgery, Cleveland Clinic Lerner College of Medicine,
Cleveland, OH

Bruce Schirmer, MD
Stephen H. Watts Professor of Surgery, University of Virginia,
Charlottesville, VA

Benjamin E. Schneider, MD
Harvard Medical School, Department of Surgery, Beth Israel
Deaconess Medical Center, Boston, MA

Kuldeep Singh, MBBS, MBA, FACS
Department of Surgery, St. Agnes Hospital, Highland, MD

Daniel E. Swartz, MD
Department of Surgery, Bariatric Program, Saint Agnes Medical
Center, Fresno, CA

Samuel Szomstein, MD, FACS
Clinical Assistant Professor of Surgery, NOVA, Southeastern
University, Associate Director, The Bariatric and Metabolic Institute,
Division of Minimally Invasive Surgery, Cleveland Clinic Florida,
Weston, FL

Steven Teich, MD
Clinical Assistant Professor of Surgery, The Ohio State University,
Department of Pediatric Surgery, Nationwide Children's Hospital,
Columbus, OH

Gonzalo Torres-Villalobos, MD
Advanced Laparoscopic Surgery Fellow, University of Minnesota,
Department of Surgery, University of Minnesota Medical Center,
Minneapolis, MN

Shawn Tsuda, MD
Department of Surgery, Beth Israel Deaconess Medical Center,
Boston MA

Olga N. Tucker, MD, FRSCI
Department of Minimally Invasive Surgery, Cleveland Clinic Florida,
Weston, FL

Mitchell S. Wachtel, MD
Associate Professor, Texas Tech University Health Sciences Center,
Lubbock, TX

Gavitt A. Woodard, BS
Stanford University School of Medicine, Stanford, CA

Rami R. Zanoun, BS
MS-II, University of Pittsburgh, Pittsburgh, PA

I. Essentials of Bariatric Surgery

1. The Rationale for Bariatric Surgery

Xingxiang Li, Orit Kaidar-Person,
and Raul J. Rosenthal

A. Introduction

The aim of these guidelines is to systematically review the clinical effectiveness of the various bariatric surgical procedures and support bariatric surgeons and allied physicians in the provision of high-quality care for morbidly obese patients.

Obesity is a serious worldwide health problem. It has been shown to predispose to various diseases, particularly cardiovascular disease, diabetes mellitus, sleep apnea, and osteoarthritis. Studies have shown that obesity is an important independent risk factor for morbidity and mortality from coronary disease; consequently, the American Heart Association continues to emphasize the importance of obesity as a major modifiable risk factor in the treatment of coronary artery disease. In the United States, the mortality rate from obesity exceeds 400,000 patients a year, and obesity is considered to be the second cause of preventable death after cigarette smoking. The long-term implications of obesity are detrimental to patients' health and are costly. It is estimated that the annual cost spent on the treatment of obesity and obesity-related health problems exceeds $100 billion. Despite various pharmacological treatments, diets, exercise, and behavioral therapy, most patients regain all lost weight within a period of 2 years.

Obesity is a disease in which the natural energy reserve, stored as fat, is increased to a point where it compromises the patient's state of being. The etiology of obesity is multifactorial, and is related to genotypic and environmental factors. Environmental factors such as social and cultural aspects, in association with genotypic factors, cause the abnormal physiology, metabolism, and behavioral and psychological pathways that result in the obesity phenotype.

The definition and classification of obesity is primarily based on the body mass index (BMI), calculated as weight divided by the square of height, by means of kilograms per square meter as the unit of measurement. Body mass index provides a reliable indicator of the level of fat in the body for most people (but not athletes), and is used to screen for weight categories that may lead to health problems. For example, Caucasians with a BMI of 30–35 kg/m² is considered as class 1 obesity, 35–40 kg/m² as class 2, and >40 kg/m² as class 3. Morbid obesity is usually defined as a BMI ≥40 kg/m² or a BMI ≥35 kg/m² in patients with comorbidities. In addition, in some cases, patients are defined as suffering from super- and mega-obesity, if their BMI >50 or 70 kg/m², respectively. Alternatively, absolute or relative increase in body weight may be used to define obesity.

Morbid obesity is a debilitating disease; it imposes physiological–psychological stress and is often associated with social isolation, depression, and other psychological and somatic comorbidities. These include metabolic complications (type II diabetes, fatty liver, cholelithiasis and hyperlipidemia), hypertension, ischemic heart disease, arthritis and respiratory system complications (obesity-hypoventilation syndrome and sleep apnea syndrome). Other common comorbidities include joint degeneration, endocrine disorders including sex hormone secretion disorders, vein congestion, and deep vein thrombosis. Disturbingly, obesity has been ignored for decades, although there is considerable evidence that suggests that obesity plays an important role in cancer pathogenesis. Obesity has been clearly associated with increased risks for kidney cancer in both genders, and in endometrial cancer and postmenopausal breast cancer in women. Studies suggest that obesity and overweight also are related to increase risk of colorectal cancer and gall bladder cancer. Obesity and overweight are often associated with gastric-reflux disease; thus, obesity may play an important role in the increasing incidence of esophageal cancer. Obesity as a predisposing factor for thyroid cancer and prostate cancer is still under evaluation.

In a recent study, the association between different grades of obesity and the number of life-years lost indicated that life expectancy is up to 20 years shorter in severe obesity. The World Health Organization (WHO) considers obesity to be the fifth major unhealthful dangerous factor because it brings inestimably potential health problems. Therefore, awareness and aggressive intervention are imperative in order to improve the patients' well-being.

B. Treatment Selection and Indications for Surgery

Weight reduction should be an integral part of any treatment regimen. Studies have confirmed that obesity is far more complex than overindulgence. These patients usually suffer from a complex disorder with genetic, metabolic, hormonal, psychosocial, and perhaps central nervous system disturbances. What is more troubling is that the pathogenesis of this disease is poorly understood and varies from patient to patient, making conventional treatment options more complicated and often unsuccessful. Weight loss can be achieved by various measures, such as nutritional modification, exercise, drugs, and bariatric surgery. Bariatric surgery has been found in numerous studies to be the most efficacious long-term treatment option for weight reduction, resulting in improvement or complete remission of comorbidities.

Surgical therapy should be considered for individuals with a BMI >40 kg/ m^2 or a BMI ≥35 kg/m^2 and significant comorbidities, in accordance with the National Institute of Health (NIH) consensus criteria for morbid obesity updated by the American Society for Metabolic and Bariatric Surgery (ASBS) in 2002.

C. Surgical Treatment: Benefit and Risk

The number of procedures continues to increase exponentially. This dramatic growth resulted from increased patient acceptance, which can be attributed in part to the introduction of laparoscopic surgery, as well as major progress achieved in other vital areas, such as anesthesia, critical care, and parenteral nutrition. Performing major surgery such as Roux-en-Y gastric bypass by laparoscopy has offered patients significant advantages, such as less pain, fewer wound complications, and early recovery with relatively low complication rates.

There are a variety of surgical options, which can be classified into the following three categories: restrictive procedures, malabsorptive procedures, and combined restrictive/malabsorptive procedures.

Restrictive procedures limit the patient's ability to take in food, but do not directly interfere with the normal digestive process. In contrast, malabsorptive procedures promote weight loss by interrupting the digestive process, causing food to be poorly digested and absorbed. Some purely malabsorptive operations are no longer recommended due to their potential to cause nutritional deficiencies. Reduced energy intake is a common goal of all procedures. Bariatric procedures can be done either by the open or laparoscopic method. Each type of bariatric procedure has associated benefits, drawbacks, and risks. The possible benefit and risk of each procedure should be carefully considered to accommodate individual patient needs and preferences. Consultation with other specialists regarding surgical options and potential risks of surgery may be appropriate. The surgeon should be quite familiar with all past and present procedures as well.

Bariatric surgery, as any other surgical procedure, carries the potential for serious morbidity and mortality. Obese patients are considered at high risk for complications in part due to the presence of significant comorbidities. Any surgical procedure performed on this population is difficult, and is often associated with technical problems related to their unusual anatomy, resulting in peculiar situations when administering drugs, positioning, and more. General anesthesia also imposes a great risk for these patients—especially patients with obstructive sleep apnea or those with symptomatic gastroesophageal reflux and other predisposing conditions—due to the increased risk for both pulmonary gastric aspiration and difficult airways. Thus, severely obese patients necessitate a multidisciplinary evaluation prior to surgery.

Complications may be classified in relation to the operative procedure (intraoperative, early, and late postoperative). The most common causes of postoperative morality include unrecognized anastomotic leak, deep vein thrombosis (DVT) with secondary pulmonary embolism (PE), and cardiac and pulmonary complications.

Early postoperative complications (<30 days) include bleeding, anastomotic leak, infection secondary to leak, strictures, anastomotic obstruction, and small bowel obstruction. Late complications (≥30 days) include ulcers, stricture, obstruction, nutritional deficiency, internal/incisional hernia, redundant skin, failure of weight loss or regain, and psychological complications.

Psychological side effects include increased depression and disruption of social relationships, and may result from unrealistic expectation from surgery and exacerbation of preoperative physiological pathology. Thus, meticulous physiological screening and informative preoperative consultation are imperative for successful outcomes.

Relative and absolute contraindications for weight loss surgery include but are not limited to high risk for cardiac complications, poor myocardial reserve, significant chronic obstructive airways disease or respiratory dysfunction, noncompliance with medical treatment, significant psychological disorders, or significant eating disorders.

Several studies have attempted to identify risk factors associated with postoperative bariatric surgery mortality. These studies have generally found preoperative weight, male gender, age, and surgeon experience to predict increased mortality risk. Comorbidities, including diabetes mellitus and hypertension, have also been identified as preoperative predictors of increased postoperative risk. The risk–benefit ratio for the aforementioned group is complicated, as patients with these pathologies often have the greatest potential to benefit from weight loss.

As Centers for Medicare and Medicaid Services (CMS) consensus regarding Medicare coverage for new bariatric surgical interventions continues to evolve, further studies may be necessary to reach a conclusion about the risks and benefits of bariatric surgery in obese patients with BMIs between 28 and 35 kg/m^2.

The increase in adult morbid obesity is becoming a major cause of death and disability in the United States and coincides with an increase in adolescent morbid obesity and the development of adult-like comorbidities. Studies show that 50–77% of obese children and adolescents carry their obesity into adulthood, with an increase in risk to 80% if there is at least one obese parent. Currently available literature provides limited data regarding the pharmaceutical and surgical treatment of obesity in adolescent and pediatric patients. The existing data on adults may be inapplicable based on the unique needs and selection criteria of the adolescent patient population. Nevertheless, behavior and lifestyle interventions for adolescent obesity have limited success as in adults, and it is unreasonable to expect adolescents with severe obesity to become normal-weight adults. In addition, obese teens experience related comorbidities with high frequency and severity. Thus, recommendations regarding bariatric surgery for adolescents have been proposed by multidisciplinary teams and published. A recent report of a multicenter study of Roux-en-Y gastric bypass outcomes at 1 year in 30 morbidly obese adolescents demonstrated excellent weight loss and resolution of comorbidities, as in adults. The frequency of complications was similar to that seen in adults. The small sample, however, precluded clear delineation of the frequency of complications. Further studies are necessary to confirm this initial favorable experience in the adolescent population.

D. Global Credentialing Requirements

To meet the global credentialing requirements in bariatric surgery, the applicant should have credentials at an accredited facility to perform gastrointestinal and bariatric surgery.

Documentation that the surgeon is working within an integrated program for the care of the morbidly obese patient that provides ancillary services such as specialized nursing care, dietary instruction, counseling, support groups, exercise training, and psychological assistance is needed. Experience in diagnosing, managing, monitoring and treating short- and long-term complications is essential for successful outcomes. The trainee should participate in follow-up visits and should either be directly supervised by the bariatric surgeon of record or other health care professionals who are appropriately trained in perioperative management of bariatric patients and part of an integrated program. Although applicants cannot guarantee patient compliance with follow-up recommendations, they should demonstrate evidence of adequate patient education regarding the importance of follow-up as well as adequate access to follow-up.

E. Experience in Bariatric Surgery Required to Train Applicants

For the purposes of this document, experienced bariatric surgeons serving as trainers for applicants should meet global credentialing requirements and have experience with at least 200 bariatric procedures in the appropriate category of procedure in which the applicant is seeking privileges prior to training the applicant.

F. Summary

Morbid obesity is a significant health concern. Medical management usually fails to achieve sustained weight loss, and medical management of obesity-related morbidities remains expensive and largely ineffective. Currently, bariatric surgical procedures are the most effective means to achieve significant, sustained weight loss, and thereby provide effective and durable treatment of obesity-associated morbidities. Experience and training in weight loss surgery, advanced surgical skills, and a commitment to long-term patient care are required for successful treatment of these patients.

G. Selected References

American Society for Bariatric Surgery. Guidelines for granting privileges in bariatric surgery. Obes Surg 2003;13:238–240.

Charuzi I, Ovnat A, Peiser J, et al. The effect of surgical weight reduction on sleep quality in obesity-related sleep apnea syndrome. Surgery 1985;97(5):535–538.

Cottam DR, Mattar S, Lord J, et al. Training and credentialing for the performance of laparoscopic bariatric surgery. Laparosc SLS Rept 2003;2(1):15–21.

Fernandez AZ Jr, DeMaria EJ, Tichansky DS, et al. Multivariate analysis of risk factors for death following gastric bypass for treatment of morbid obesity. Ann Surg 2004;239(5):698–702.

Fernandez AZ Jr, DeMaria EJ, Tichansky DS, et al. Experience with over 3,000 open and laparoscopic bariatric procedures: multivariate analysis of factors related to leak and resultant mortality. Surg Endosc 2004;18(2):193–197.

Flum DR, Dellinger EP. Impact of gastric bypass operation on survival: a population-based analysis. J Am Coll Surg 2004;199(4):543–551.

Flum DR, Salem L, Elrod JA, et al. Early mortality among Medicare beneficiaries undergoing bariatric surgical procedures. JAMA 2005;294(15):1903–1908.

Gastrointestinal surgery for severe obesity: National Institutes of Health Consensus Development Conference Statement. Am J Clin Nutr 1992;55:615S–619S.

Herrera MF, Deitel M. Cardiac function in massively obese patients and the effect of weight loss. Can J Surg 1991;34:431–434.

Hu FB, Manson JE, Stampfer MJ, et al. Diet, lifestyle, and the risk of type 2 diabetes mellitus in women. N Engl J Med 2001;345:790–797.

Livingston EH, Huerta S, Arthur D, et al. Male gender is a predictor of morbidity and age a predictor of mortality for patients undergoing gastric bypass surgery. Ann Surg 2002;236(5):576–582.

McGoey BV, Deitel M, Saplys RJ, et al. Effect of weight loss on musculoskeletal pain in the morbidly obese. J Bone Joint Surg Br 1990;72(2):322–323.

Mun EC, Blackburn GL, Mathews JB. Current status of medical and surgical therapy for obesity. Gastroenterology 2001;120:669–681.

Nguyen NT, Ho HS, Palmer LS, et al. A comparison study of laparoscopic versus open gastric bypass for morbid obesity. J Am Coll Surg 2000;191(2):149–155.

Oliak D, Ballantyne GH, Weber P, et al. Laparoscopic Roux-en-Y gastric bypass: defining the learning curve. Surg Endosc 2003;17(3):405–408.

Schauer P, Ikramuddin S, Gourash W, et al. Outcomes after Laparoscopic Roux-en-Y gastric bypass. Ann Surg 2000;232:515–529.

Wittgrove AC, Clark GW. Laparoscopic gastric bypass, Roux-en-Y- 500 patients: technique and results, with 3–60 month follow-up. Obes Surg 2000;10(3):233–239.

Wolfe BM, Morton JM. Weighing in on bariatric surgery: procedure use, readmission rates, and mortality. JAMA 2005;19;294(15):1960–1963.

2. Overview of Bariatric Operations

Daniel E. Swartz and Edward L. Felix

A. Overview of Bariatric Surgery

Overweight, obesity, and morbid obesity, defined as body mass indices greater than or equal to 25, 30, and 40 kg/m², respectively, constitute a burgeoning global epidemic. Approximately 30% of Americans are obese, of whom over 5 million suffer from morbid obesity. For the latter cohort, bariatric surgery is the only effective means to achieve significant weight loss with improvement or resolution of comorbid diseases. The field of bariatric surgery began over 50 years ago and has grown steadily and, over the last decade, explosively, with over 100,000 procedures performed annually in the United States.

The purpose of this chapter is to present the reader with a framework for understanding the numerous described bariatric surgical procedures along with their historical development. The evolution of these operations has not been a linear process, as previously abandoned procedures have been modified and re-introduced. As newer technologies emerge, this framework will permit the reader to compare their function, advantages, and limits of use to existing procedures.

Bariatric operations are classified as purely malabsorptive, purely restrictive, or combined malabsorptive-restrictive (Fig. 2.1). An additional category, entitled "miscellaneous," contains the procedures that do not fit into the three standard classes. Note that no distinction between "laparoscopic" or "open" procedures is made, since these are merely approaches to perform a given procedure. The advantages of a laparoscopic approach (less pain, faster recovery, and fewer wound-related complications) are well established and require no further discussion here. The bariatric surgeon requires a thorough understanding of the recognized operations and, based on his or her ability, may perform them utilizing a laparoscope or a laparotomy.

B. Purely malabsorptive procedures

Purely malabsorptive procedures were initially popular in the 1960s and 1970s. Because of the risk of vitamin and protein deficiencies as well as diarrheal issues, these procedures are no longer performed as primary bariatric surgery in the United States.

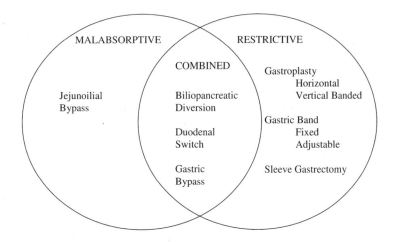

Figure 2.1. Venn diagram of the recognized bariatric operations.

1. Jejunoileal bypass

a. Development. The first surgical procedure performed on a large scale to treat obesity was the jejunoileal bypass (JIB). Early animal studies began at the University of Minnesota in 1953 and led to the first published clinical series by Kremen in 1954, who performed an end-to-end jejunoileostomy with drainage of the bypassed bowel into the colon. Severe complications and early failures led to the development of the classic 14-4 end-to-side jejunoileostomy.

b. Technique. The proximal jejunum is divided 14 inches (35.5 cm) from the ligament of Treitz and anastomosed to the terminal ileum 4 inches (10 cm) proximal to the ileocecal valve (Fig. 2.2).

c. Outcome. Approximately 25,000 patients have undergone a JIB. Patients achieved roughly 50% of excess body weight loss (EBWL). Malabsorptive side effects were significant, with severe electrolyte, nutrient and vitamin deficiencies; protein-energy malnutrition with alopecia and liver failure; renal oxalate urolithiasis from intestinal binding of dietary calcium by fatty acids; polyarthropathy by circulating immune complexes from bacterial proliferation and absorption in the bypassed limb; and socially impairing profuse and foul-smelling diarrhea from malabsorption of fat.

d. Current status. This operation has been abandoned since the early 1980s and most of the patients are thought to have been reversed or revised to other procedures. Our knowledge of intestinal malabsorption and, in particular, bypass enteritis has been significantly advanced from this procedure. Today, all bariatric procedures have intestinal limbs through which pass either food or bile so as to avoid the blind loop.

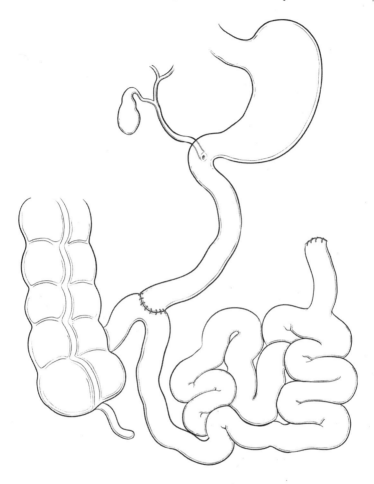

Figure 2.2. Jejunoileal bypass.

C. Combined Restrictive–Malabsorptive Procedures

1. Biliopancreatic diversion

a. Development. Scopinaro first described this procedure in 1979, which was designed to enhance the benefits of a malabsorptive procedure while minimizing the profile of side effects. Although the procedure involves a hemigastrectomy, leaving a 250- to 500-ml pouch, the restriction of this procedure is limited as the stomach stretches, and the long-term weight loss and comorbidity resolution is attributed to the significant malabsorption. Distal gastrectomy is essential so as not to leave an intact antrum leading to uninhibited gastrin secretion with marginal ulcer formation, otherwise known as the "retained antrum syndrome." Adequate pouch size is similarly essential in order to counteract protein and macronutrient malabsorption by increasing intake. Scopinaro hypothesized that direct contact of undigested food with the ileal mucosa is thought to cause early satiety and, in the initial postoperative period, mild discomfort and vomiting; a state referred to as the "post-cibal syndrome."

b.   Technique. Distal gastrectomy including the pylorus is performed, leaving a 250- to 500-ml proximal gastric pouch. The ileum is divided 250 cm proximal to the ileocecal valve and the distal stump is anastomosed to the gastric pouch. The proximal stump (biliopancreatic limb) is anastomosed to the distal ileum 50 cm from the ileocecal valve (Fig. 2.3).

c.   Outcome. Two large series of patients with 15-year follow-up demonstrated approximately 71% EBWL regardless of preoperative BMI and co-morbidity resolution that was equal or superior to results following gastric bypass. Morbidity occurs in 30%, including protein-energy malnutrition in 12.6%, ulcers in 8.3%, and a perioperative mortality of 1.3%.

d.   Current status. The BPD achieves excellent weight loss and comorbidity resolution even in the superobese; however, mortality and long-term morbidity rates that exceed other bariatric procedures have tempered the enthusiasm for this procedure in North America. Most surgeons who advocated a preference for the BPD have migrated in favor of the duodenal switch (see the following).

2. Duodenal switch

a.   Development. DeMeester first described this surgery in 1987 to treat bile reflux; however, Hess and Hess are credited with the first series of the duodenal switch (DS) to treat obesity in 1988. The DS has been lauded as a safer alternative to the BPD, with less malabsorption (and hence fewer malabsorptive sequelae), greater restriction, less marginal ulceration, less dumping, and lower perioperative mortality.

b.   Technique. A sleeve gastrectomy is performed leaving a 200-ml gastric reservoir with the pylorus included in the alimentary limb. The duodenum is divided just distal to the pylorus and anastomosed to the ileum 250 cm proximal to the ileocecal valve. The biliopancreatic limb is then anastamosed to the ileum 100 cm from the ileocecal valve (Fig. 2.4).

c.   Outcome. The 100-cm common channel of the DS has led to significantly fewer malabsorptive complications, such as fewer bowel movements per day and lower incidence of iron, calcium, and vitamin A deficiency when compared with BPD. Percent EWL is approximately 73% at 4 years, which is roughly equivalent to BPD.

d.   Current status. Most surgeons who once advocated for BPD have migrated to the DS camp. Overall this represents a minority of North American bariatric surgeons. Since the weight loss in the superobese (BMI > 50) exceeds that found in Roux-en-Y gastric bypass, some

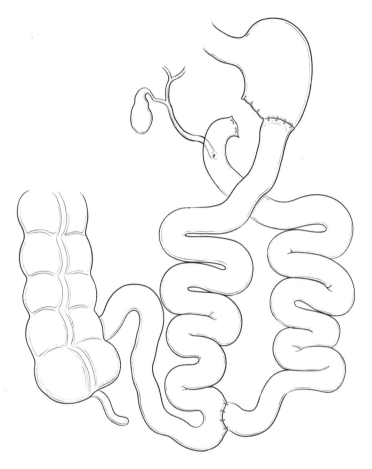

Figure 2.3. Biliopancreatic diversion.

surgeons have advocated for this technique in this group of patients either as a single- or two-staged procedure. Others have performed DS as a secondary procedure following other failed bariatric operations.

3. Gastric bypass

a. Development. Mason and Ito are credited with the first gastric bypass (GBP) for morbid obesity in 1966. Their operation included a horizontal gastric pouch with a 100- to 150-ml reservoir anastomosed to a loop of jejunum. This operation has evolved over the last four decades into what is considered the gold standard bariatric procedure to which all other procedures are compared. The fundamental modifications

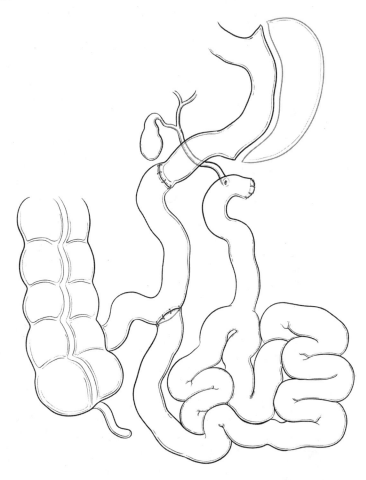

Figure 2.4. Duodenal switch.

included a Roux-en-Y drainage, vertical pouch based on the less-distensible lesser curvature, isolated gastric pouch (divided from the gastric remnant) with less than 30-ml volume and a 10- to 15-mm anastomosis. Brolin randomized superobese patients (BMI > 50) to 75 vs. 150 cm alimentary (Roux) limb lengths and found significantly improved excess weight loss at 2 years (50% vs. 64%, respectively).

b. Technique. The gastric pouch is created by creating a 15- to 30-ml pouch based on the lesser curve by stapling either "free-hand" or around a 32–34 French gastric lavage tube or Baker balloon. Care is taken to avoid injury to the left gastric artery, which supplies the pouch, and to exclude the fundus by not dividing the stomach to the left of the angle of His. The proximal jejunum is divided and the distal stump (alimentary limb) is brought antecolic, retrocolic antegastric, or retrocolic retrogastric and anastomosed to the gastric pouch to create a 10- to 12-mm diameter stoma. The proximal stump of jejunum (biliopancreatic limb) is anastamosed to the alimentary limb either 75 to 100 cm distal to the gastrojejunostomy (BMI < 50) or 150 cm (BMI ≥ 50) (Fig. 2.5).

c.   Outcome. Similar to the BPD and DS, the GBP results in dramatic metabolic and weight changes but with fewer malabsorptive sequelae. Excess body weight loss varies from 60% to 75% for 10 years and 50% at 14 years. Reported rates for comorbidity resolution are diabetes (80%), hypertension (70%), hypercholesterolemia (65%), gastroesophageal reflux disease (75%), and obstructive sleep apnea syndrome (75%). Thirty-day perioperative mortality is 0.5%. Potential vitamin and mineral deficiencies from malabsorption requiring lifelong monitoring include iron, calcium, folic acid, and vitamin B_{12}. The most severe complications include leaks (0–3%), internal herniation with or without strangulated bowel obstruction (2–5%), and perforated marginal ulcer (1%). Less severe complications include anastomotic stenosis (5–10%). Perioperative (30-day) mortality rates are 0.2% to 1% in most recent published series; however, larger regional surveys have reported up to 2%.

d.   Current status. The GBP is the most commonly performed bariatric surgery, accounting for 85% of procedures in the United States and 65% worldwide. This is due to its excellent and durable results with low morbidity and mortality rates.

D. Purely Restrictive Procedures

1. Gastroplasty

a.   Development. The gastroplasty procedures were an attempt to create a safer more physiologic procedure without intestinal anastomoses where leaks may occur. The stapled gastroplasties in which a partial partition was made by either horizontally or vertically placed staples to create a restrictive gastric pouch. However, the staple lines tended to break down with complete loss of restriction. Various modifications were described without success until Mason's series on vertical banded gastroplasties (VBGs) in 1982. This procedure utilized a restrictive pouch based on the lesser curvature with multiple staple lines and a stoma reinforced with prosthetic mesh.

b.   Technique. A 32-French bougie is placed via the mouth and advanced along the lesser curve. An EEA stapler anvil is passed full thickness through the stomach from the lesser sac approximately 5 cm distal to the gastroesophageal junction. Several applications of a TA-90 or similar stapler are fired vertically to the left of the bougie across the angle of His. The stoma is then reinforced with a band of prosthetic material (Fig. 2.6).

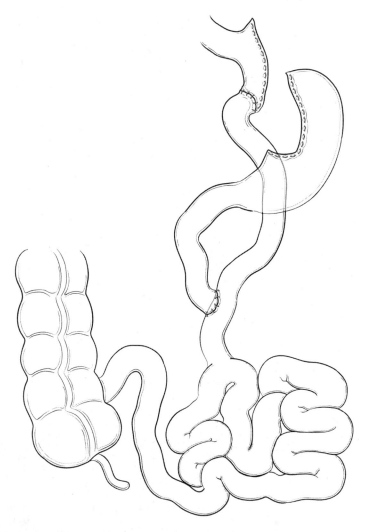

Figure 2.5.   Roux-en-Y gastric bypass.

c.   Outcome. Morbidity and perioperative mortality rates were low (10%
and 0.25%) and patients achieved 35% to 60% EBWL during the first
year, but many patients regain significant weight over the long term.
Staple-line dehiscences with marginal ulcerations as well as stomal
stenoses with reflux were commonly encountered.

d.   Current status. The gastroplasty procedures have been largely abandoned given their long-term failures and high rates of requiring
revisional procedures.

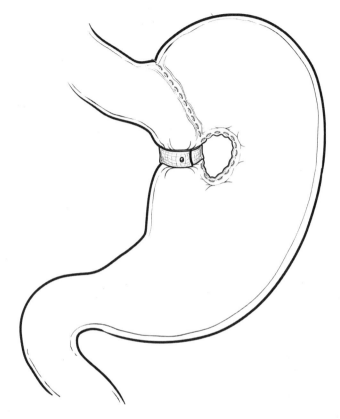

Figure 2.6. Vertical banded gastroplasty.

2. Gastric banding

a.   Development. Gastric banding procedures are the least invasive, have
     the lowest propensity for vitamin and nutrient deficiencies, and have
     the lowest morbidity and mortality among bariatric operations. With the
     advent of the adjustable band using a subcutaneous port, this procedure
     has become the most commonly performed bariatric operation in Aus-
     tralia and parts of Europe. Nonadjustable prosthetic material wrapped
     around the proximal stomach over a Nissen fundoplication was first
     described by Wilkinson in 1981, and 2 years later Bo described the
     first placement of a gastric band. Kuzmak introduced the adjustable
     gastric band (AGB) connected to a Port-A-Cath–type self-sealing res-
     ervoir placed in the subcutaneum in 1990. Currently performed on an
     outpatient basis or 24-hour stay, these bands induce satiety by exerting

a constant, gentle pressure on the proximal gastric wall that leads to a dramatic reduction in appetite and food intake. In order to be effective, the procedure requires regular outpatient adjustments and a patient who is highly disciplined in avoiding energy-dense liquids. Initial rates of complications such as posterior gastric prolapses and erosions reported with the perigastric technique through the lesser sac have been markedly reduced using the pars flaccida technique.

b.   Technique. Minimal dissection is the key as the gastrophrenic ligament is dissected sufficiently to safely pass a blunt instrument posterior to the fundus. The pars flaccida of the gastrohepatic ligament is divided to expose the right crus. A small window through the phrenoesophageal ligament along the right crus is made to pass a blunt instrument through the retrogastric tissue to create a tunnel just large enough to pass the band. The tubing is passed through the buckle, where it is fastened and anterior gastrogastric sutures are placed to create an anterior tunnel to prevent anterior prolapses. The tubing is externalized where it is connected to the subcutaneously placed port (Fig. 2.7).

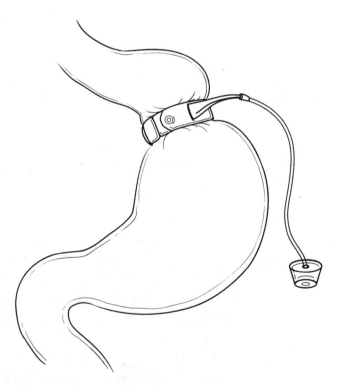

Figure 2.7.   Gastric band—adjustable.

c. Outcome. Weight loss following AGB is gradual, reaching 50–60% EWL by 3 years, which remains stable over periods up to 7 years. The US experience, however, has been more variable, with higher failure rates and band explantations. Resolution of medical comorbidities is good but generally does not attain the superior results of the GBP, BPD, or DS. The most severe complications include gastric prolapse, or "band slippage," in up to 5%, and band erosion in 0% to 1%. However, tube breakages, leaks, and port problems requiring surgical correction occur in 10% to 15%. Perioperative mortality is 0.05%.

d. Current status. The AGB is the preferred procedure in Australia and parts of Europe, accounting for 30% of bariatric surgeries worldwide and 15% in the United States. Long-term data demonstrate that this procedure is effective and durable. The AGB is a good option for the motivated patient willing to comply with a postoperative adjustment schedule of every 4 to 6 weeks in the initial year and who understands that the weight loss is gradual over 3 years.

3. Sleeve gastrectomy

a. Development. The sleeve gastrectomy (SG), in which a narrow tubular stomach is created based on the lesser curvature with resection of greater curvature gastric remnant, is the first part of the DS procedure, as previously described. Due to presumed increased morbidity and mortality with superobese patients undergoing RYGB or DS, Regan proposed a staged procedure in which an SG is performed first and then converted to a DS or GBP after a period of initial weight loss. This "initial weight loss" turned out to be substantial, with 50% to 60% EWL over 12 months and, combined with a favorable safety profile, the SG has lately been proposed as a definitive stand-alone bariatric procedure.

b. Technique. The greater omentum and gastrocolic ligament are separated from the greater curvature of the stomach beginning at a point 2 to 3 cm from the pylorus and extending proximally to include division of the gastrosplenic ligament with the short gastric vessels. A 32- or 34-French bougie is advanced along the lesser curvature and the stomach is divided with linear staplers around the bougie from a point on the greater curvature 2 to 3 cm from the pylorus to the angle of His.

c. Outcome. In a meta-analysis of 15 studies, 12-month %EWL was 51 (45–81) with 9% complications, including bleeding and staple-line leaks and a perioperative mortality of 0.6%. Many of these studies included primarily higher risk patients with greater BMIs.

d. Current status. The SG has been touted as both an initial stage of another bariatric procedure, such as a DS or GBP, as well as a stand-alone operation. Recent reports of using the SG as a definitive procedure demonstrate impressive weight loss and comorbidity improvement with low morbidity and mortality for high-risk patients at 12 months but long-term effects are currently unknown.

E. Miscellaneous Procedures

1. Jaw wiring

Maxillomandibular fixation (MMF) is a temporary method to prevent over-feeding using orthodontic devices with wires. Although this procedure was more popular in the last century, it is still offered by some practitioners. The wires need to be removed for several days every 4 to 6 weeks to prevent stiffness and they are rarely left in place beyond 6 months. They have been shown to induce a moderate degree of weight loss in some patients the weight usually returns once it is removed. Wire cutters need to be carried at all times in case of emergencies such as vomiting or choking. With the established safety, effectiveness, and durability of other bariatric procedures for even the larger, higher-risk patient, there is little benefit to be obtained by MMF.

2. Intragastric balloon

Endoscopic placement of an intragastric balloon filled with 400 to 700 ml of fluid has seen resurgence in popularity in recent years. Like MMF, it is a temporary procedure with a strict recommendation to remove it within 6 months. Weight loss during this period has been reported up to 33% EWL, with complete weight regain following deflation if a definitive bariatric procedure does not ensue. Patients at high risk for a definitive surgery may improve their risk profile with an initial substantial weight loss, but complications such as obstruction, gastric perforation, and death have been reported. The intragastric balloon is at present only investigational in the United States.

3. Implanted gastric pacemaker

Electrical impulses to induce gastroparesis and anorexia serve as the impetus for the implanted gastric pacemaker (IGP). Cigaina reported these results in animal studies in which an implanted pacemaker that stimulated the lesser curvature of the stomach between the gastroesophageal junction and pylorus. Clinical trials are few but the largest experience comes from Europe, where morbidly obese patients underwent placement of the IGP. At 1- and 2-year follow-up, % EWL was 20 and 25, respectively, with minimal morbidity. At this time, the IGP is solely experimental.

F. Summary

After half a century of growth and development, bariatric surgery is still an array of procedures in evolution. The application of the laparoscope along with improvements in safety and a dramatic reduction in morbidity and mortality has made these procedures more acceptable to patients. Despite their popularity, the large volume of bariatric operations performed has not kept pace with the epidemic rise in obesity rates worldwide.

The armamentarium of procedures to treat obesity attests to the lack of a single ideal surgical remedy. As further refinements are made and new technologies become available, we will undoubtedly see even greater and more durable weight loss, better outcomes for comorbidities, and enhanced safety profiles. This brief overview of existing procedures will hopefully provide the reader a framework in which to evaluate current treatments and integrate future ones.

G. Selected References

Belachew M, Legrand M, Vincent V, et al. Laparoscopic adjustable gastric banding. World J Surg 1998;22:955–963.

Bo O, Modalsli O. Gastric banding, a surgical method of treating morbid obesity: preliminary report. In J Obes 1983;7:493–499.

Brolin RE, Kenler HA, Gorman JG, et al. Long-limb gastric bypass in the superobese: a prospective randomized study. Ann Surg 1992;215:387–395.

Brolin RE, Kowalski C. Operations for morbid obesity. In: Yeo CJ, Dempsey DT, Klein AS, et al. editors. Shackleford's surgery of the alimentary tract, 6th ed. Philadelphia: Saunders/Elsevier, 2007:928–939.

Cigaina V, Pinato G, Rigo V, et al. Gastric peristalsis control by mono situ electrical stimulation: a preliminary study. Obes Surg 1996;6:247–249.

De Csepel J, Quinn T, Pomp A, et al. Conversion to a laparoscopic biliopancreatic diversion with a duodenal switch for failed laparoscopic adjustable silicone gastric banding. J Laparoendosc Adv Surg Tech A 220;12:237–240.

DeMeester TR, Fuchs KH, Ball CS, et al. Experimental and clinical results with proximal end-to-end duodenojejunostomy for pathologic duodenogastric reflux. Ann Surg 1987;205:414–426.

Doherty C. Vertical banded gastroplasty. Surg Clin N Am 2001;81:1097–1112.

Griffen WO, Young VL, Stevenson CC. A prospective comparison of gastric and jejunoileal bypass operation for morbid obesity. Ann Surg 1977;186:500–507.

Gumbs AA, Gagner M, Dakin G, et al. Sleeve gastrectomy for morbid obesity. Obes Surg 2007;17:962–969.

Hess DS, Hess DW. Biliopancreatic diversion with duodenal switch. Obes Surg 1988;8:267–282.

Keshishian A, Zahriya K, Hartoonian T, et al. Duodenal switch is a safe operation for patients who have failed other bariatric operations. Obes Surg 2004;14:1187–1192.

Kremen AJ, Linner LH, Nelson CH. An experimental evaluation of the nutritional importance of proximal and distal small intestine. Ann Surg 1954;140:439–448.

Kuzmak LI. Surgery for morbid obesity. Using an inflatable gastric band. AORN J 1990;51:1307–1324.

MacLean LD, Rhode BM, Sampalis J, et al. Results of the surgical treatment of obesity. Am J Surg 1993;165:155–162.

Marceau P, Hould FS, Simard S, et al. Biliopancreatic diversion with duodenal switch. World J Surg 1998;22:947–954.

Marinari GM, Murelli F, Camarini G, et al. A 15-year evaluation of biliopancreatic diversion according to the Bariatric Analysis Reporting Outcome System (BAROS). Obes Surg 2004;14:325–328.

Mason EE. Vertical banded gastroplasty for obesity. Arch Surg 1982;117:701–706.

Mason EE. Why the operation I prefer is the vertical banded gastroplasty 5.0. Obes Surg 1991;1:181–183.

Mason EE, Ito C. Gastric bypass in obesity. Surg Clin N Am 1967;47:1345–1351.

O'Brien PE, Dixon JB. Laparoscopic adjustable gastric banding in the treatment of morbid obesity. Arch Surg 2003;138:376–382.

Poiries WJ, Swanson MS, MacDonald KG, et al. Who would have thought it? An operation proves to be the most effective therapy for adult-onset diabetes mellitus. Ann Surg 1995;222:339–350.

Regan JP, Inabnet WB, Gagner M, et al. Early experience with two-stage laparoscopic Roux-en-Y gastric bypass as an alternative in the super-super obese patient. Obes Surg 2003;13:861–864.

Schauer P. Gastric bypass for severe obesity: approaches and outcomes. Surg Obes Rel Dis 2005;1:297–300.

Scopinaro N, Adami GF, Mariari GM, et al. Biliopancreatic diversion. World J Surg 1998;22:936–946.

Scopinaro N, Gianetta E, Civalleri D. Biliopancreatic bypass for obesity: II. Initial experience in man. Br J Surg 1979;66:618–620.

Slater GH, Fielding GA. Combining laparoscopic adjustable gastric banding and biliopancreatic diversion after failed bariatric surgery. Obes Surg 2004;14:677–682.

Torres JC, Oca CF, Garrison RN. Gastric bypass: Roux-en-Y gastrojejunostomy from the lesser curvature. South Med J 1983;76:1217–1221.

Wilkinson LH, Peoloso OA. Gastric (reservoir) reduction for morbid obesity. Arch Surg 1981;116:602–605.

3. Identification of Comorbidities and Their Management

Benjamin E. Schneider

A. Introduction

Weight loss surgery (WLS) has become accepted as a treatment for obesity and many of its comorbidities. Current indications for WLS require that patients with a body mass index between 35 and 40kg/m^2 suffer from severe comorbid disease in order to attain insurance coverage for surgery. Obesity associated diseases including sleep apnea, diabetes, hypertension, cholelithiasis, thrombophlebitis, and pulmonary embolus may all affect surgical morbidity and mortality. Preoperative identification of existing comorbidities may be necessary in order to secure access to surgical therapy and enable care givers to intervene in order to optimize outcomes.

B. Obstructive Sleep Apnea

The incidence of sleep apnea in patients undergoing WLS may be 35% to 77%. Patients undergoing WLS frequently exhibit characteristics concerning for obstructive sleep apnea (OSA) such as BMI greater than 35kg/m^2, increased neck circumference, nasal obstruction, micrognathia, macroglossia, snoring, frequent nocturnal arousal from sleep, and somnolence.

OSA has been associated with pulmonary hypertension, stroke, hypertension, cardiac ischemia, dysrhythmia, and sudden death. Preoperative diagnosis and treatment of OSA may reduce hypoxia/hypercarbia, reduce airway mucosal edema, reduce pulmonary shunting, and potentially improve surgical outcomes. Patients undergoing WLS should be evaluated with overnight polysomnography if suspected of moderate to severe sleep apnea. In patients with diagnosed sleep apnea, either CPAP or BiPAP should be instituted preoperatively. Ideally, patients will bring their own CPAP/BiPAP equipment with them on the day of surgery as this is generally better tolerated following anesthesia. The perioperative anesthetic approach to patients with OSA includes judicious use of narcotic and benzodiazepines, elevation of the head during intubation and extubation, and extubation when the patient is fully awake. Postoperatively, patients should be monitored for airway obstruction and hypoxia.

C. Cardiovascular Disease

It is predictable that some measure of cardiovascular dysfunction is relatively common among patients undergoing WLS given the incidence of metabolic syndrome, hyperlipidemia, hypertension, diabetes, peripheral vascular disease, and sleep apnea in the severely obese. Generally patients undergoing WLS are stratified by American Heart Association guidelines as intermediate risk. All patients should undergo an electrocardiogram and have a review of a recent lipid panel. The clinical history and exam should help delineate those patients in whom poor functional status, cardiac risk predictors, or symptoms necessitate further cardiac testing. Subsequent evaluation with either a dobutamine stress echo or nuclear stress testing may then help identify patients requiring a referral to a cardiologist. A previous history of rheumatic fever or use of diet pills (e.g., phentermine-fenfluramine) should undergo an echocardiogram to assess for valvular disease. Although lacking in high level evidence and recently more controversial, consideration should be given to the use of β-blockers.

D. Deep Vein Thrombosis

Among the medical conditions associated with morbid obesity are venous insufficiency and thrombosis. Obesity is associated with derangements in coagulation, which may lead to hypercoagulability. Preoperative assessment should focus upon patient characteristics, including history of thromboembolic events, venous stasis/insufficiency, smoking, oral contraceptive use, sleep apnea, age, and hypercoagulable states. Generally we advise patients to refrain from smoking and oral contraception for 8 weeks prior to surgery. Unless otherwise contraindicated mechanical as well as either unfractionated or low-molecular-weight heparin should be employed perioperatively. In patients at highest risk consideration may be given to preoperative placement of an inferior vena cava filter.

E. Type 2 Diabetes

Among comorbidities, type 2 diabetes has the strongest link with obesity; 80% of type 2 diabetics are obese. Screening of patients prior to WLS is important as half of type 2 diabetics are previously undiagnosed. Routine screening should include fasting plasma glucose and glycosylated hemoglobin (HbA1C). Patients diagnosed with diabetes should have their blood glucose controlled prior to surgery. HgA1C reflects the degree of glycemic control over the erythrocyte life span (120 days) generally should be <9%.

F. Liver Disease

In addition to diabetes and central obesity, nonalcoholic fatty liver disease (NAFLD) is an established consequence of metabolic syndrome. As the global epidemic of obesity has grown, the incidence of NAFLD has risen to estimates as high as 25%. The clinical spectrum of the disease ranges from relatively benign steatosis to nonalcoholic steatohepatitis (NASH), the latter of which may progress to cirrhosis. NASH may progress to fibrosis in 25% to 30% of cases.

Preoperatively patients should be screened with liver function testing, platelet count, coagulation panel, and serum albumen. Serum aminotransferase levels and bilirubin are not completely sensitive, as values may be normal in the setting of severe disease. Advanced fibrosis and inflammation should be suspected in patients with an AST/ALT ratio of greater than 1. A liver ultrasound may demonstrate a bright-hyperechogenic parenchyma, hepatomegaly. Doppler may be helpful in assessing hepatic and portal vein flow. Preoperative weight loss may improve ALT levels and liver size. Intraoperative liver biopsy should be considered in patients with hepatic dysfunction, metabolic syndrome, or gross liver disease.

G. Cholelithiasis

The incidence of cholelithiasis among morbidly obese patients may be 45%, as compared with 10% to 20% in the general population. Furthermore, an increase in the incidence of gallstones following weight loss is well described. This led surgeons to advocate for cholecystectomy at the time of WLS, particularly in the case of malabsorptive procedures in which rapid weight loss is achieved. Sugerman (1995) described the routine use of prophylactic ursodiol in order to reduce the risk of stone formation following gastric bypass surgery. While uniform standards do not exist for routine screening with ultrasound either preoperatively or intraoperatively, it is our practice to attempt to identify patients with gallstones. Patients may then be counseled as to appropriate management.

H. Selected References

Dixon JB. Surgical treatment for obesity and its impact on NASH. Clin Liver Dis 2007;11:86–101.

Gross JB et al. Practice guidelines for the perioperative management of patient with obstructive sleep apnea. Anesthesiology 2006;104:1081–1093.

Saltzman E, et al. Criteria for patient selection and multidisciplinary evaluation and treatment of the weight loss surgery patient. Obes Res 2005;13:234–243.

4. Definition of Obesity and Indications for Surgery

Jamie D. Adair and Mark A. Pleatman

A. Indications

Obesity is an excess of body fat that frequently results in a significant impairment of health. It is a chronic, lifelong, genetically related, life-threatening disease of excessive fat storage. Obesity results when the size or number of fat cells in a person's body increases. A normal-sized person has 30 to 35 billion fat cells. When a person gains weight, these fat cells first increase in size and later in number. One pound of body fat represents about 3,500 calories. The prevalence of overweight and obesity in the United States make obesity a leading public health problem that can have medical, social, psychological, and economic consequences. Obesity is growing at an exponential rate: It is estimated that there are more than 150,000 bariatric operations performed each year in the United States.

Although "overweight" technically refers to an excess of body weight and "obesity" to an excess of fat, these two words can be defined operationally in terms of body mass index. The body mass index (BMI) is the most practical way to evaluate the degree of obesity, although it does not take into account the different ratios of adipose to lean tissue. Visceral fat (or central obesity) has a much stronger correlation with certain diseases, such as cardiovascular disease, than the BMI alone. The absolute waist circumference (>102 cm in men and >88 cm in women) or waist–hip ratio (>0.9 for men and >0.85 for women) are both used as measures of central obesity.

Another way to determine obesity is to assess the percent of body fat but this can be a little challenging and often requires specialized equipment. The most accurate measures are to weigh a person underwater or to use an X-ray test called dual energy X-ray absorptiometry (DEXA). It is generally agreed that men with more than 25% body fat and women with more than 30% body fat are considered obese.

Bariatric surgeons use the BMI when evaluating candidates for potential bariatric surgery. It is calculated from the height and weight as follows:

$$BMI = \text{body weight (in kg)} \div \text{square of stature (height, in meters)}$$

For example, a man who is 5′ 10″ (1.78 meters) tall and weighs 285 lbs (135 kg) would have a BMI of $130/1.78 \times 1.78 = 41$.

Overweight is defined as a BMI between 25 and 30 kg/m^2 and obesity as a BMI greater than 30 kg/m^2. The current definitions commonly in use establish the following values, agreed in 1997 and published by the WHO in 2000 are summarized in the following:

- A BMI less than 18.5 is *underweight*
- A BMI of 18.5–24.9 is *normal weight*
- A BMI of 25–29.9 is *overweight*
- A BMI of 30–39.9 is *obese*
- A BMI of equal to or greater than 40 is *severely (or morbidly) obese*

The latest estimates are that around 30% of adults in the United States are obese and 5% are considered morbidly obese. Morbid obesity (or clinically severe obesity) is recognized as a major public health risk throughout the world, and has been clearly shown to reduce life expectancy. Certain comorbid conditions associated with obesity are largely responsible for the mortality and morbidity of this disease. Cardiac disease, diabetes mellitus type II, obstructive sleep apnea, hypertension, dyslipidemia, gastroesophageal reflux disease, stress urinary incontinence, arthritis of the weight-bearing joints, infertility, and some cancers have all been linked to obesity (Table 4.1). Bariatric surgery has proven to be an effective means to aid in the management of these comorbidities. The previous chapter deals with the identification of these comorbid conditions and their management.

B. Indications for Operation

Medical management alone has a high failure rate to sustain greater than 10% weight loss in obese patients; and management of comorbidities is often expensive and insufficient. The surgical treatment of morbid obesity has been well established as being safe and effective. In addition, the short-term and long-term improvement in comorbidities has been well documented. Surgery should be only one part of a long-term multidisciplinary approach that should include monitoring for nutritional and metabolic complications and dietary counseling to prevent weight gain. Psychological and behavioral factors as well as an assessment of perioperative risk and complications must be considered before bariatric surgery. For these reasons, the NIH in 1991 issued a consensus statement and acknowledged that "alone, objective clinical features is not sufficient to make a decision regarding surgery." Although each potential surgical case should be assessed for risks and benefits, the consensus statement offered the following guidelines for patient selection:

- Patients should have a low likelihood of responding to traditional, non-surgical therapy. Often, these patients have previously tried medically sound weight loss programs without success.

Table 4.1. Comorbidities associated with obesity.

Hypertension	Certain carcinomas	Venous stasis
Cardiovascular dysfunction	Sexual hormone dysfunction	Degenerative arthritis
Respiratory insufficiency	Infectious complications	Pseudotumor cerebri
GERD	Hyperlipidemia	Psychosocial impairment
Diabetes	Heart disease	Chronic lower back pain
Skin disorders	Gout	Sleep apena
Asthma	Urinary stress incontinence	

- Patients must be well informed and motivated and accept the operative risks. They also need to be able to participate in and comply with treatment and follow-up.
- Patients should have a BMI in excess of 40kg/m^2 or body weight greater than 100 lbs above ideal body weight.
- Patients are candidates if they have a BMI between 35 and 40kg/m^2 along with more than one high-risk comorbid condition or body weight greater than 80 lbs above ideal body weight with a comorbidity.
- An important conclusion of the 1991 National Institutes Consensus Development Conference Statement on the surgical treatment of obesity was that "patients judged by experienced clinicians to have a low probability of success with non-surgical measures, as demonstrated, for example, by failure in established weight control programs or reluctance by the patient to enter such a program, may be considered for surgical treatment."

The Society of American Gastrointestinal Endoscopic Surgeons (SAGES) therefore recommends that surgical therapy should be considered for individuals who:

Have a body mass index (BMI) of greater than 40kg/m^2
OR
have a BMI greater than 35kg/m^2 with significant comorbidities
AND

can show that dietary attempts at weight control have been ineffective

The indications for laparoscopic treatment of obesity are the same as for open surgery.

Guidelines in the past also recommended that patients should be over the age of 18 or under 60 years of age. There is not a lot of literature with regard to these patients undergoing bariatric surgery, but a recent study indicates that it may be safe for some of these individuals.

There are certain contraindications for bariatric surgery, including: no medical management attempted, life-threatening diseases, lack of social support, inability to follow up, substance abuse, and patients who have psychiatric disorders that have been evaluated by a psychiatrist.

C. Selected References

Cowan GSM Jr, Hiler ML, Buffington CK. Criteria for selection of patients for bariatric surgery. In: Deitel M, Cowan GSM Jr, eds. Update: surgery for the morbidly obese patient. Toronto: FD Communications, 2000:161–170.

Gastrointestinal surgery for severe obesity. Proceedings of a National Institutes of Health Consensus Development Conference. March 25–27, 1991, Bethesda, MD. Am J Clin Nutr 1992;55:487S–619S.

Hazzan D, Chin EH, Steinhagen E, et al. Laparoscopic bariatric surgery can be safe for treatment of morbid obesity in patients older than 60 years. Surg Obes Relat Dis 2006;2:613–616.

Health Implications of Obesity. NIH Consensus Development Conference Statement. Ann Intern Med 1985;103:1073–1077.

Kellum JM, DeMaria EJ, Sugarman H. The surgical treatment of morbid obesity. Curr Probl Surg 1998;35:796–851.

Mun EC, Blackburn GL, Mathews JB. Current status of medical and surgical therapy for obesity. Gastroenterology 2001;120:669–681.

Ogden CL, Carroll MD, Curtin LR, et al. Prevalence of overweight and obesity in the United States, 1999–2004. JAMA 2006;295:1549–1555.

Peeters A, Barendregt JJ, Willekens F, et al. Obesity in adulthood and its consequences for life expectancy: a life-table analysis. Ann Intern Med 2003;138:24–32.

World Health Organization. WHO technical report series 894: Obesity: preventing and managing the global epidemic. A Report of a WHO Consultation. Geneva, 2000.

5. Preoperative Nutritional Assessment and Postoperative Dietary Guidelines

Andrew B. Lederman

A. Preoperative Nutritional Assessment

Nutritional assessment is an essential part of the patient evaluation prior to weight loss surgery. Morbidly obese patients often have clinical or subclinical nutritional deficiencies. Although the morbidly obese patient has an excess store of fat, there may be deficiencies in protein or micronutrients. This may be due to baseline eating habits or poorly managed efforts at weight loss. Preoperative deficiencies, if left untreated, may worsen after weight loss surgery, and subclinical deficiencies may manifest into significant illness with potentially devastating consequences.

1. Common preoperative deficiencies

Common preoperative deficiencies include low levels of protein, vitamin D (25-OH), thiamine, iron, and folate.

a. **Protein** deficiencies preoperatively are usually related to diet and may raise the risk of complications with surgery. Deficiency may worsen after surgery due to dietary restriction and/or malabsorption.

b. **Vitamin D** deficiency may commonly be found preoperatively. Since increased bone turnover may be a concern after RYGB, vitamin D levels should be corrected if low prior to surgery. **Calcium** deficiency can be associated with malabsorptive procedures, and may exacerbate osteopenia.

c. Body stores of **thiamine** last a relatively short 6 to 8 weeks, so preoperative deficiencies may quickly develop after surgery, with potentially devastating neurologic consequences.

d. **Iron** deficiency, and related anemia, is common, especially in women of childbearing age. Since iron is predominantly absorbed in the duodenum, deficiencies may worsen after surgery.

e. B_{12} and **folate** are less often a problem before surgery, but postoperative diet restriction and malabsorption may lead to decreased levels and subsequent anemia. Assessment of preoperative levels may be useful for following levels after surgery.

f. **Vitamin A** deficiency has been associated with obesity, although not as commonly as other micronutrients. Postoperative deficiency has been seen with malabsorptive procedures. Both reversible and irreversible sequelae have been seen with postoperative vitamin A deficiency.

g. Other micronutrients or vitamins, such as **copper**, **zinc**, **selenium**, **niacin**, **biotin**, **vitamin B$_6$**, and fat-soluble vitamins **E** and **K** are rarely deficient preoperatively, but may become problematic after surgery. Since deficiencies are less common, serum levels are not routinely measured prior to surgery unless a baseline is desired for postoperative comparison.

2. Role of the dietitian

Consultation with a registered dietitian or nutritionist prior to surgery is required of all patients. This encounter should include an assessment of current eating habits, including behaviors and food choices, the calculation of postoperative nutritional goals, and the education of the patient on how to reach these goals. The dietitian may also help with preoperative weight loss should it be needed.

3. History and physical exam

A complete history and physical exam may identify signs of nutritional deficiency. Eating habits, food preferences, and diet history are part of a complete history. Physical findings of chronic rash, poor wound healing, or hair loss may all be signs of pre-existing deficiency.

4. Laboratory evaluation

Serum levels are the best way to assess the different elements of nutrition, and are an important part of the preoperative evaluation. Protein nutrition should be evaluated by **prealbumin** and **albumin. Thiamine, folate, 25-OH vitamin D, iron**, and **ferritin** should all be checked. **Calcium** and parathyroid hormone should be checked if vitamin D levels are low or the patient is known to have osteopenia. **Prothrombin time** should be measured if vitamin K is a concern. Levels of vitamin B$_{12}$, vitamin A, zinc, selenium, niacin, biotin, and copper may be useful preoperatively as a baseline for postoperative follow-up.

Preoperative deficiencies should be corrected with supplementation.

B. Postoperative Nutritional Guidelines

Nutritional requirements after weight loss surgery will vary with the type of procedure, the degree of malabsorption, and the patient. Specific diets and the progression from one to the next may vary among programs. However, some general guidelines can be followed.

1. Caloric goals

Most postoperative diets focus on achieving appropriate levels of protein and limiting empty sources of calories. The restriction provided by weight loss procedures such as gastric bypass, gastric banding, and sleeve gastrectomy limits the volume that can be eaten, but this effect may wane over time, and a caloric goal may be useful to help patients limit their intake. For most patients, caloric intake should range from 1,000 to 1,400 kcal/day.

2. Protein

Dietary protein is essential to safe and effective weight loss. Most postoperative diets aim for a daily protein intake of 40 to 60 g/day. Patients with BPD may require 60 to 90 g/day due to the greater malabsorption of that operation.

Early after surgery, many patients use high-protein supplements to reach their protein goal. Many high-protein supplements are also high in calories, and these should be avoided. Protein shakes should be consumed as meals, not sipped throughout the day, since that may lead to excessive intake of either calories or protein.

As patients progress toward a more regularly textured diet, they should strive to achieve their protein goal via dietary sources. Appropriate sources of protein include low-fat dairy products, beans, poultry, eggs, fish, and soy. Lean meats are also acceptable. A typical day might include four servings of dairy (approximately 1/2 cup) and four servings of another protein source each day to reach the protein goal.

The early satiety associated with restrictive procedures can limit protein intake. Patients should be encouraged to eat protein first with each meal and avoid beverages immediately prior or during meals. This prevents them from reaching satiety prior to consuming their protein.

3. Carbohydrates and simple sugars

Carbohydrates and simple sugars should make up only a small portion of the diet. Patients should be limited to one to two small servings of carbohydrates each day, with 1/4 cup of mashed potatoes considered to be one serving. Diets should provide about 50 g of carbohydrates each day, with milk, fruit, vegetables, and starches as appropriate sources of carbohydrates.

Patients on an extremely low carbohydrate diet may develop ketosis. This is common in the early postoperative period when patients are on a full liquid or puréed diet and it is harder to achieve 50–100 g/day of carbohydrates.

Simple sugars should be avoided as empty calories and as stimuli for dumping syndrome. In general, a portion needs to have less than 10 g of simple sugars to avoid dumping syndrome. Some sugars, such as fructose, glucose, and galactose, tend to be better tolerated than sucrose or high-fructose corn syrup.

Sugar substitutes, such as aspartame, saccharin, or sucralose, may be used. Sugar alcohols such as sorbitol may not be well tolerated.

4. Fats

Fats should be taken sparingly, but are essential. Most recommendations are for 25 g/day or less. Fatty acids are required for absorption of fat-soluble vitamins, and essential fatty acids such as arachidonic acid can only be obtained from dietary sources. Fats should preferably be omega-3 fatty acids found in fish, canola oil, and flax seed. Polyunsaturated fats from vegetable oils and saturated fats from animal fats and coconut oil should be avoided.

5. Vitamins, minerals, and supplements

Patients will all require vitamin supplementation after surgery. A daily multivitamin is recommended for all weight loss surgery patients. This will provide maintenance levels of vitamins A, D, E, and K, thiamine, folate, niacin, riboflavin, vitamin B6, vitamin C, folate, and vitamin B_{12}.

Additional supplementation is based upon postoperative serum levels and other risk factors. Menstruating women may require iron supplementation in the form of ferrous sulfate at 45 to 60 mg/day. Postmenopausal women are at a high risk of osteoporosis with weight loss, and should be on calcium citrate with vitamin D at 500 mg three times each day.

All patients with malabsorptive procedures should have vitamin B_{12} supplementation, in the form of 1,000 mcg/month intramuscularly, 100 to 1,000 mg/day orally, 500 to 1,000 mg weekly sublingually, or 500 mg each week as a nasal spray.

Combination vitamins that include variable amounts of vitamin B_{12}, intrinsic factor, iron, vitamin C, and folate (i.e., Conison, Foltrin, Trinsicon, and Fergon Plus) are available and are both effective and convenient for treating several deficiencies.

Hair loss in the setting of adequate protein intake may indicate deficiencies of zinc, selenium, or biotin. Zinc sulfate 200 mg/day or zinc gluconate 30 to 50 mg/day is acceptable. Selenium supplementation is usually 50 to 100 mcg/day. Biotin is available as part of a good B-complex vitamin or can be taken 300 to 600 mg/day if needed.

Folate, thiamine, niacin, vitamins A, E, K, C, B_6, and riboflavin are usually adequate with a daily multivitamin. These micronutrients and trace elements such as copper should be followed with serum levels. In the setting of a specific deficiency each can be supplemented appropriately.

6. Postoperative diet progression

Most programs use a progression of diets after surgery. These diets are usually designed to be low in calories, high in protein, and low in carbohydrates and fats. The diets restrict the texture of food to allow the stomach and any anastomosis to heal.

a. **Full liquid diet** uses liquid meals that are separate and distinct from any beverages consumed during the day to maintain hydration.

b. **Pureéd** or **blended diet** allows a thicker consistency, but no large chunks of food. Food should be the consistency of applesauce or thinner.

c. **Soft foods** are fork-tender, and need to be well chewed before swallowed. Raw vegetables, red meat, or other tough foods are excluded. Bread or other soft foods that form a firm bolus when chewed and swallowed should also be avoided.

d. The last stage incorporates **regular textured foods**. This allows foods of any consistency, as long as they are low fat, low calorie, low carbohydrate, and high protein. The exception may be fibrous or sticky foods that may cause difficulty with the stoma of a LAGB.

7. Eating behaviors

Modification of preoperative eating habits is critical to postoperative success and avoiding complications. Patients need to be taught and encouraged to follow some simple rules:

a. **Eat only at regularly scheduled times.** This usually means three small meals each day, with two small snacks during the day.

b. **Eat slowly** and **chew food well.** Food should be chewed to the consistency of a liquid.

c. Patients should **eat protein first** so that early satiety does not limit protein intake.

d. Avoid drinking during meals and for 30 minutes before and after meals. Beverages near meal times can cause enough satiety that it can be difficult to get adequate amounts of protein.

e. **Measure portions** to avoid overeating. Using a small salad plate rather than a dinner plate helps maintain small portions. Patients have a tendency over time to slowly increase their portion size, which may lead to weight regain.

f. Stop when satiety is reached.

g. **Avoid sticky or fibrous foods.** This can be particularly important for LAGB patients. Foods such as asparagus or celery may block the stoma of an adjustable gastric band. Sticky foods such as reheated rice or pasta can cause similar problems.

C. Selected References

Flancbaum L, Belsley S, Drake V, et al. Preoperative nutritional status of patients undergoing Roux-en-Y gastric bypass for morbid obesity. J Gastrointest Surg 2006;10:1033–1037.

Kuruba R, Koche LS, Murr MM. Preoperative assessment and perioperative care of patients undergoing bariatric surgery. Med Clin North Am 2007;91:339–351.

Parkes E. Nutritional management of patients after bariatric surgery. Am J Med Sci 2006; 331(4):207–213.

Tucker ON, Szomstein S, Rosenthal RJ. Nutrition consequences of weight loss surgery. Med Clin North Am 2007;91:499–514.

6. Essentials of a Bariatric Program

Troy A. Markel and Samer G. Mattar

A. Introduction

The obesity epidemic continues to grow at an alarming rate. As the number of weight loss operations grows exponentially, so does scrutiny on the outcomes of these complex procedures. Such oversight has led to the recognition that surgical outcomes in morbidly obese patients are optimized through a detailed evaluation of the patient, and the ability to provide a wide range of services at all stages of management. Such thorough and holistic management can only be delivered through a comprehensive weight loss program that includes a variety of components that synergistically address all aspects of the care of the morbidly obese patient.

This chapter briefly discusses the components of a comprehensive bariatric program, including essential staff, support programs, material infrastructure, and education. The successful integration of these components is essential in making the results of weight loss surgery both safe and durable.

B. Facilities

Bariatric offices should be attractive and appealing. Patient acquisition and retention will be enhanced by providing furnishings and room plans that not only accommodate every patient, but also positively signal that these patients are welcome and strongly desired. This philosophy should commence at the initial surgeon's practice, and continue throughout all aspects of patient care, including within other consultant offices, as well as within hospital facilities.

Programs specializing in bariatric care should have oversized chairs in waiting areas and patient exam rooms. In addition, specialized examination tables with hydraulic lift capabilities are essential for assisting patients in appropriately positioning them for a physical examination. Scales for weighing patients, as well as all additional medical equipment, including blood pressure cuffs, should be of an adequate size to provide appropriate measurements. Patient gowns and other clothing articles should be large and accommodating, and readily available in all examination rooms.

In the hospital, patient beds should have the weight capacity to safely bear morbidly obese patients. In addition, they should be appropriately constructed to prevent bed sores or injury. Operating rooms should be spacious, and all surgical equipment must be compatible with larger patients. It is imperative that operating room staff be familiar with the limitations of all equipment, and be able to follow alternative arrangements if patients exceed those limitations. Adequate restroom facilities, including wide stalls and shower facilities, as well as commodes that are affixed to the floor as opposed to the wall, are an essential accommodation in any bariatric program. Finally, all doors and wheelchairs should be wide enough to allow for easy patient access and transport.

C. Personnel

1. Nurse coordinator and bariatric nurse

A nurse, who may also occupy the position of program coordinator, is an essential member of any bariatric program. It is important that patients be evaluated by a skilled professional who is familiar with the physical and psychological characteristics of the morbidly obese patient. Many postoperative patients experience a variety of symptoms that may be effectively managed by a skilled nurse. The bariatric nurse should occupy a central position in any program, and should play a pivotal role in facilitating interactions between patients and other staff members, and communicate with hospital staff regarding specific patient requirements.

2. Dietician/nutritional consultants

There is a growing recognition that bariatric surgeons are essentially metabolic surgeons. Bariatric surgeons are assuming this role as a result of the profound metabolic consequences of restrictive or malabsorptive weight loss procedures. Although the majority of these effects are beneficial, there is potential for negative outcomes due to nutritional deficiencies, some of which may be lethal. For these reasons, as well as many others, it is imperative that skilled nutritionists be available who have a deep understanding of the special feeding characteristics of morbidly obese patients and the nutritional challenges they face.

At the first encounter, nutritionists evaluate the patients' eating patterns and meal proportions, and carefully analyze their relationship with food. This evaluation often influences the development of special preoperative dietary plans that prepare the patient for the expected changes and challenges of weight loss surgery. In the postoperative period, many patients often have no appetite, sometimes for the first 6 months or more. Most bariatric postsurgical patients have to adhere to a schedule for eating since they will not be prompted by hunger.

Nutritionists and dieticians also counsel postoperative patients on the appropriate food items and quantity of foodstuffs to consume. Proteins are the most important food source as they allow for appropriate maintenance of muscle tissue. Nutritionists advise patients on food sources with high protein content, and on appropriate chewing and swallowing techniques. Patients and their families also need to be made aware of the dumping syndrome, which often accompanies operative procedures that bypass the duodenum. Patients should be instructed to avoid high carbohydrate foods, particularly those that also contain a high proportion of fats, such as chocolate and pastries.

The daily administration of vitamin and nutrient supplementation is critical after any weight loss surgery, and it is the incumbent responsibility of the surgeon to ensure that patients maintain adequate vitamin and nutrient balance. The most frequent nutrient aberrations involve iron, B_{12}, calcium, and vitamin D. Calcium losses and low vitamin D levels are common after bariatric procedures, and active supplementation is required to prevent the sequelae of secondary hyperparathyroidism.

3. Psychologists

Although many bariatric programs outsource their psychological evaluations, active counselors are an integral part of any successful weight loss program. Psychologists offer invaluable support in assessing patients' mental conditions, and frequently counsel patients to withstand the lifelong changes associated with surgical weight loss procedures. Counselors aid patients in allaying the apprehensions of weight loss, and guide them in obtaining healthy perspectives of self-image. It is important that patients have a realistic expectation of the rate of weight loss, as many patients may feel that weight loss will occur immediately after surgery. In addition, although outcome predictors are not completely understood, it is well recognized that patient knowledge, psychosocial adaptation, and motivational factors are important in achieving successful weight loss after bariatric surgery.

4. Surgeon

Physicians who perform surgical weight loss procedures should have in-depth training within the field of general surgery, as well as comprehensive training in bariatric and minimally invasive procedures. The learning curve is steep; therefore, some form of advanced training is recommended. Although a bariatric fellowship is not required for clinical privileges, many surgeons who anticipate having a high volume of bariatric procedures may choose to undergo a 1-year fellowship that specializes in bariatric and minimally invasive surgery. However, many practicing surgeons are unable to interrupt their practices to dedicate an entire year to specialized training. Our studies have indicated that providing carefully designed mini-fellowship programs to practicing general surgeons in the form of a 6-week minimally invasive bariatric fellowship provides adequate exposure for these physicians to competently perform surgical weight loss procedures.

Ultimately the surgeon is responsible for the entire comprehensive bariatric care service, and he or she should be involved in the immediate and long-term postoperative care of the bariatric patient. A structured follow-up plan is essential to ensure the continued effectiveness of the weight loss procedure. With time, the medical supervision of bariatric patients may be transferred to other physicians, such as bariatricians, or perhaps the patients' primary physicians, provided they adhere to the recommended follow-up outline as set up by the bariatric program.

5. Anesthesiologist

Morbidly obese patients often have multiple medical comorbidities, and may suffer substantial and severe limitations in physiologic reserve. Anatomical limitations due to thick necks and crowded oral cavities may pose additional anesthetic challenges. Such circumstances raise the anesthetic risk and require the presence of skilled and experienced anesthesiologists. Special anesthetic equipment and ventilators capable of generating high pressures are required to overcome the mass effect of body habitus. The volume of distribution of some medications may also be altered based on the proportion of fat tissue. All these factors dictate the need for anesthesiologists who are familiar with the safe perioperative management of this high-risk population.

D. Education and Support

1. Educational seminars

Patients considering bariatric surgery will undoubtedly benefit from preoperative educational seminars. Patients gain an acquaintance to the overall scheme of the program, including the staff, the pathway they will follow in the preoperative evaluation, the characteristics of the various bariatric procedures, the expected postoperative course, and the dietary changes that are required should they participate in a surgical weight loss procedure. Emphasis is placed on the need for lifelong follow-up and periodic assessment of nutritional parameters.

The educational seminars are usually 1 to 2 hours in duration, and preferably involve presentations by the surgeon and other program staff, supplemented with appropriate audiovisual aids and printed materials for future review. Patients are encouraged to bring their family members to these sessions, and both patients and their family should be given ample opportunities to ask questions in order to understand the surgical options and follow-up plans.

2. Support group meetings

Support group sessions are designed to promote discussion among patients regarding appropriate expectations for weight loss and progression toward healthy living. Discussions should be moderated by a health care professional with familiarity of the challenges and changes that bariatric patients face. These sessions are primarily intended for postoperative patients and their families, but should also be attended by preoperative patients who may be considering weight loss surgery. Topics for discussion should be broad and free-spirited, but always controlled and monitored for realistic and appropriate content. An actual schedule of future topics adds an educational flavor to these meetings, and occasional lay presentations by clinical experts are enthusiastically received by patients.

3. Social programs

Many comprehensive bariatric programs promote fun and educational activities for their patients. Postoperative activities may include exercise programs and social outings. In addition, cooking classes are often held onsite to show patients how to prepare healthy foods. These classes are often combined with educational workshops by the nutritionists, and serve to promote healthy eating habits. In addition, a variety of exercise programs that involve weight training and cardiovascular activities promote physical activity in the long-term postoperative period.

4. Electronic resources

Due to the proliferation of the internet, potential bariatric patients are able to research weight loss surgery from numerous sources. This concept may be beneficial, but with the plethora of information available, patients also have access to erroneous information. Therefore, it is advised that comprehensive bariatric programs invest in creating a dedicated electronic resource. Such a web site should contain an explanation of the problems associated with obesity, as well as the potential medical and surgical solutions to these problems. All information should be presented in lay terms, and should describe the organization of the program, as well as the preoperative and postoperative pathways that patients will follow. Additionally, patients may submit a basic application form electronically via the web site, so that staff could prescreen patients prior to attending the educational seminar. Chat rooms for patients, as well as an area where patients could directly contact the members of the care team, may provide a means of communication that is more effective and efficient than traditional telephone communication.

It is also imperative for bariatric centers to maintain a database of information that includes patient demographics and comorbidities, as well as operative procedures, postoperative complications, and follow-up results. A comprehensive database that links all bariatric centers will provide valuable information for both clinical and research purposes. In addition, a well-maintained database will allow the care team to analyze past performances, complication rates, and other parameters that will allow them to improve the care provided to their patients.

E. Conclusion

As the rate of obesity continues to rise, and the beneficial outcomes of weight loss surgery continue to be recognized, there will be increasing demand on surgeons to safely and effectively treat patients. Since obesity is a disease that affects patients globally, it makes intuitive sense to treat these patients through a comprehensive bariatric care team. Led by the surgeon, this team should be able to effectively evaluate prospective patients and prepare them mentally and physically for the profound behavioral changes associated with surgery. Such a comprehensive team needs talented and dedicated personnel, a strong infrastructure, and most importantly, a pervasive philosophy that morbid obesity is a chronic disease process that can be effectively treated within the confines of a comprehensive bariatric surgical program.

F. Selected References

Benotti P, Wood GC, Still C, et al. Obesity disease burden and surgical risk. Surg Obes Relat Dis 2006;2(6):600–606.

Cottam D, Holover S, Mattar SG, et al. The mini-fellowship concept: a six-week focused training program for minimally invasive bariatric surgery. Surg Endosc 2007;21(12):2237–2239.

Markel TA, Mattar SG. Management of gastrointestinal disorders in the bariatric patient. Med Clin North Am 2007;91(3):443–450.

Mattar SG, Rogula T. Essentials of a Bariatric Surgery Program. In: Sugarman HJ, Nguyen N, eds. Management of morbid obesity. New York: Taylor & Francis, 2006:61–73.

Poitou Bernert C, Ciangura C, Coupaye M, et al. Nutritional deficiency after gastric bypass: diagnosis, prevention and treatment. Diabetes Metab 2007;33(1):13–24.

Pratt GM, McLees B, Pories WJ. The ASBS Bariatric Surgery Centers of Excellence program: a blueprint for quality improvement. Surg Obes Relat Dis 2006;2(5):497–503, discussion.

Tucker ON, Szomstein S, Rosenthal RJ. Nutritional consequences of weight loss surgery. Med Clin North Am 2007;91(3):499–514, xii.

7. Psychological Assessment

Eldo E. Frezza, Mitchell S. Wachtel, and Rolf Gordhamer

A. Introduction

Although it would seem logical for the "eating public" to grasp the reality of the obesity epidemic and to appropriately diet, emotional obstacles to successful weight loss are monumental. Eating is a stress reliever, a friend, a pacifier, and a companion on lonely nights. Eating until stuffed, for many, numbs floating anxiety, helping sufferers to cope with the general existential angst of modern life. Before undergoing bariatric surgery, emotional elements must be assessed and treated to ensure a successful outcome. This chapter outlines our approach to determining whether a patient is psychologically appropriate for weight loss surgery.

B. Checklists

1. Symptom Checklist 90

An array of tools is available to psychologists. The Symptom Checklist 90 (SCL-90), reported in Table 7.1, may or may not satisfy a particular psychologist's needs, but one can add or delete items as needed. SCL-90 has 90 items divided into nine parts each with ten items. In our experience, some reorganization proved useful to better clarify issues requiring the most emphasis.

While women check off far more areas of concern, men sometimes simply check two or three of the 90 items. When queried about any other items they might consider noting, such men usually say nothing else is relevant. This contrasts with the clinical interview, which generally reveals a traumatic history or a frustrated life.

As might be expected, the most commonly checked items relate to physical complaints, depression, and personal sensitivity. Obese persons are often in physical distress, are very conscious and insecure in public, and often are depressed. Compulsive behavior items are commonly checked. Often, two or more phobias are indicated, especially "afraid of tight places" and "feeling uneasy in crowds." In terms of paranoia, patients often indicate that they agree that they have the "feeling that you are being watched or talked about," consistent with their being hypersensitive to the glances and looks by people in crowds.

It is critical to explore any items checked that indicate psychotic thinking. Men sometimes check the item "having thoughts about sex that bother you a lot"; this generally relates to feeling rejected by women due to their weight, which can

Table 7.1. Main categories of the SCL 90.

1. Negative effect	6. Social withdrawal
2. Health problems	7. Hostility control
3. Psychotic features	8. Suicidal thinking
4. Acting out	9. Alienation
5. Anger control	10. Alcohol problems

yield hostile sexual fantasies. Occasionally checked is "the idea that something is wrong with your mind," which sometimes serves as an explanation for obesity.

C. Wahler Physical Symptoms Inventory

The Wahler Physical Symptoms Inventory (WPSI) asks about 42 physical symptoms and is quite useful as a means of assessing the range and extent of physical discomfort. This tool is very useful for evaluating a patient for hyperchondriasis. One needs to ascertain if there are more complaints than expected or beyond a typical response. Such persons can have a difficult recovery after surgery, are prone to excessively call the physician with physical concerns and postsurgical complaints, and sometimes have unrealistic expectations of the degree of relief of physical symptoms as they lose weight.

The patient reviews each of the 42 physical symptoms, rating their occurrence as: almost never (0), once a year (1), once a month (2), once a week (3), twice a week (4), or nearly every day (5). The scores are summed and divided by 42 to yield an average, which is converted into a percentage. The test is standardized, with male and female norms derived from tests of the adult population in general. The most commonly reported symptoms are back aches, numbness of body parts, muscular tension, headaches, difficulty sleeping, feeling tired, difficulty breathing, pain in the hands feet, arms, and legs, and bowel trouble. One should compare these results with those of the health problems section of the Personality Assessment Screen.

D. Personality Assessment Screen

The Personality Assessment Screen (PAS), a brief form of the Personality Assessment Inventory (PAI), which has 344 items and takes 40 to 50 minutes to complete, has 22 items in 10 personality categories, as detailed in Table 7.2. Each question is scored false (0), slightly true (1), mainly true (2), or very true (3); totals are classified as low (0–12), normal (13–15), mild (16–18), moderate (19–23), marked (24–44), and extreme (45–66). Care must be exercised if the "health problems" section totals 4 or more. Social withdrawal and alienation are frequently high. The two questions that compose the subcategory "psychotic features" are "some people do things to make me look bad" and "some people try to keep me from getting ahead"; although the PAS sees these statements as an

Table 7.2. Main categories of the PAS test.

1. Physical concerns	5. Anxiety
2. Compulsive behavior	6. Phobias
3. Personal sensitivity	7. Hostility
4. Depression	8. Psychotic thinking
	9. Paranoia

Table 7.3. Main categories of the SF-36 test.

1. Physical function
2. Physical role limitations
3. Emotional role limitations
4. Bodily pain
5. Mental health
6. General health

indication of a psychotic nature, in today's competitive office environment, they can simply reflect reality. The questions can generate hostile responses by the morbidly obese. All assessment devices have weaknesses; psychologists must be cognizant of each tool's shortcomings and take them into consideration when reaching conclusions about a client.

E. Other Assessment Tools

We have used a modified SF-36 Questionnaire (Table 7.3); our paper showed that women improved in physical functioning and mental health after bariatric surgery.

F. Formal Interview

Before interviewing the patient, the results of the checklists (SCL-90, WPSI, and PAS) are reviewed; a set of guided question is then prepared. The purposes of the interview are to: (1) ensure that the patient is free from psychological factors that may interfere with good long-term results and (2) assess the need for presurgical counseling. Patients, who usually have never seen a psychologist apart from Dr. Phil or some actor on television portraying a psychologist, enter the office with apprehension; a gentle approach is mandatory.

After reviewing insurance information, the spelling of their name, and their address, the first question is always, "Why the extra weight?" Some respond with, "What?" and a confused look, as if was the least probable question they would have been asked. Some say, "I have no idea why I'm fat. I just am," which suggests a potentially long interview to sort out the causes or factors for the obesity. Others quickly lay out a history of their life, detailing every trauma ever experienced, with an explanation of how it impacted their eating behavior. Direction is essential: One is not interested in the loss of a dog at 6 years of age or the scholastic failures of patient's children. Sometimes it is necessary to interrupt and move on to more relevant data. Another common response to, "Why the extra weight?" is, "It's genetic," which is a way of saying, "Don't blame me for the obesity." Others responses include, "I just love food," trauma (e.g., divorce, death of a child, job loss), childhood abuse, and in the case of women, repeated pregnancies.

A patient's weight history is always important. One asks about weight gain from childhood in 5- to 10-year increments, using such prompts as, "What was your weight when leaving high school?" to stimulate specific memory. Most patients are able to recall specific weights. Also important is learning if the patient ever lost what he or she considered a significant amount of weight, why this occurred, and why it was not permanent.

One then asks if eating results for stress or boredom, which almost always yields a positive response, including such things as, "I'm an emotional eater; any emotion will trigger my eating." Patients often reveal a physical injury involving their back, feet, or hip that slowed or stopped physical activity. "I used to jog or play softball but I can't anymore" is commonly expressed.

G. Family Weight

One next delves into the childhood eating milieus. How did the family deal with food? What were their attitudes toward meals? Was it a sit-down meal every night with balanced food items or run out for fast food? A vital question is, "Is anyone in your immediate family, mother, father, sisters, or brothers 80 to 100 lbs overweight?" This explores the influences at play in the family system. Usually, one hears that multiple relatives, especially siblings, are morbidly obese. Often, parents or grandparents are dying or have died of obesity-related diseases. Sometimes, one side of the family comprises obese persons. Some will even say such things as, "I want this surgery because I watched my aunt waste away from...." Families are often completely out of touch with their bodies, with a limited connection between what they put in their mouths and the state of their health.

H. Daily Food Intake

The next question is, "What is a typical day's food consumption for you?" Breakfast can be variable. Often patients can overeat so much in the evening that the morning lacks hunger. A common answer begins, "I stop for one or two breakfast burritos on the way to work." A few patients will tell about a cup of tea and piece of toast or cup of yogurt. Most patients who work face the same limited lunch options that everyone else does; lunch is often fast food on the run. A few have sit-down lunches with friends where they can special order and eat low-calorie dishes. The great dangers are: (1) the snack room and (2) the various celebrations, with caloric treats, undertaken by fellow employees to celebrate a birthday or simply to charm others with sweets. Dinner for most single patients is fast food. Those who are married with children enjoy a meal of meat, potatoes, and vegetables. When asked, most patients report eating until they are totally full. Commonly, patients have "something sweet" before bed. Some wake at 2:00 AM to snack. Others continuously snack during the day, often drinking caloric soft drinks at the same time. This information is vital to assess the barriers patients will face after surgery. A strategy is necessary; patients need to know temptation prowls and how to distract themselves and avoid situations that will defeat the purpose of bariatric surgery.

I. Obesity and the Body

The next question is, "How has the obesity affected your physical body?" Commonly reported are back pain, swelling of limbs, hypertension, exhaustion, foot pain, joint pain, diabetes, and sleep problems. When bariatric surgery is considered, patients are usually at the tail end of a battle against their bodies. Watching someone struggle with cancer or crutches, hauling 350–400 lbs into your office chair can be difficult. On some occasions, the surgical assistance is sought at the first sign of physical deterioration. Most, however, seem to be at death's door before they seek help; the patient realizes that "if I don't do something radical I will be totally incapacitated or dead." It is this thought that most often prompts a decision to seek weight loss surgery.

J. Commercial Weight Loss Systems

The next question is, "Have you tried other weight loss systems?" Almost all patients have tried a variety of the many commercial approaches available in our society. A few say, "I have tried my own system once or twice." Most people, especially women, are able to rattle off a staggering list of commercial systems they have tried, including Nutri-System, Weight Watchers, Slim-Fast, Tops, Herba Life, Opti Fast, and Dr. Atkins diet. Patients generally report some initial success but then they level off. They stray from the diet and in turn gain more weight on top of where they started.

K. Emotional Ideation: Suicidal Thinking

The next question is, "Do you have any thoughts of harming yourself?" Most patients deny this, but the psychologist must listen and observe the patient carefully, especially for a pause, which usually indicates a defensive, evasive, or dishonest response. The patient may clear their throat, or look in another direction or shift uncomfortably in the chair. In such cases, one might follow up with, "I think perhaps there is more to tell about this." Some recall past thoughts or attempts during teen years or after a traumatic event; when this occurs, one should ask for details and check how close they are to being back at that point on a scale of

1 to 10. One rarely hears about present thoughts of self-harm, but indications that these are present include that the patient was thinking about such things a month or less ago. Sometimes, thoughts of self-harm center about a specific event from which they are recovering. More worrisome are periodic suicidal thoughts without apparent trigger or event. In such cases, it is vital to learn if the patient sought professional help and suggest the acquisition of professional assistance (from a psychiatrist, psychologist, licensed professional counselor, or clinical social worker with a master's degree) if this has not been done. Some patients consider their youth counselor at the church or pastor to be adequate as a therapist; the patient must in such cases be directed to seek the advice of a licensed professional.

L. Depression

One next asks about symptoms and diagnoses made by others of depression. Many patients arrive with their depression medicines in hand for you to examine. There is emotional pain innate in weighing over 100 lbs above your recommended weight, which usually leads to spouses' avoiding intimate relations, children being embarrassed by their obese parents, and being stared at and commented upon by strangers in malls and grocery stores. Obese women particularly sense the disapproval of the general population. The obese person generally thinks poorly of themselves having let their condition get to a point of endangering their health. They are very critical of not having the will power or self-discipline to lose the extra pounds. They have experienced a long history of failure in weight loss. Most, if not all, obese persons suffer some degree of depression. When asked if the depression is weight-related or due to other circumstances, most respond by saying the depression is related to the obesity.

M. Substance Abuse

Patients in our experience usually deny alcohol, although they may report alcohol or drug use in the remote past. This may be due to our patient population, which comprises mostly middle-class persons from New Mexico and Texas with relatively strict standards of appropriate behavior; in other locales, such as large urban areas, this might be a more important issue. Our patients, when asked, also usually deny laxative abuse and bulimia. Notwithstanding this, we also routinely ask if patients have sought counseling or therapy before, the issues related to such professional care, and also if they were ever hospitalized for emotional or substance abuse issues.

N. Physical/Sexual Abuse

Childhood experiences of sexual abuse, molestation, rape, or physical abuse are vital; some women who have faced such trauma gain weight to avoid the sexual attention of men. It is common for young girls to have experienced inappropriate sexual attention from older male neighbors and relatives, often grandfathers. Not uncommon is molestation by another child. The patient often denies that the incident was significant or states that some insufficient response, such as telling their mother or attending one or two professional sessions, permitted them to "move on" from the experience.

Recently, a patient reported having been repeatedly raped by her father as a child. She neither told anyone about nor sought therapy for these incidents. The patient felt much of her obesity was related to this trauma. Because we were unsure how the patient would react to having the protective weight removed, she was referred for extensive therapy before bariatric surgery. Some female patients report physical abuse by a spouse or significant other; although the abuse was usually from an ex-husband or ex-boyfriend, it is always important to ascertain if abuse is occurring at present and take appropriate action to ensure that it stops. Although not related to abuse itself, it is always important to know if the spouse or significant other also has weight problems.

O. Supportive People

The next question is, "Who is emotionally supportive to you in this process?" It is important to uncover the attitude of the spouse, usually the husband, toward bariatric surgery. Although the usual response is, "he wants me to do what makes me happy," what is being sought for is the spouse afflicted by jealousy or insecurity. Such men can interpret bariatric surgery as an attempt to look better and find another man for herself; this can result in attempts to sabotage the results, either blatant or subtle. Of cultural interest, Hispanic men sometimes desire their wives to be obese, perhaps as an indication of commitment to the marriage. Whenever such issues are uncovered, discussions with the marriage partner are vital to ensure that the surgery will be successful. Such discussions are always of some use because the spouse, even when not insecure, will be able to learn of the adjustments that may occur in the life of the family, including dining habits, leisure habits, and socialization patterns.

Hearing that the patient's family and friends are involved is a very positive sign. Patients should be told that the end of obesity sometimes means a change in social systems. Some obese friends may no longer feel comfortable with the new improved body of the patient. The patient may be spending their time at the gym or recreation center instead of snacking in someone's living room. Sometimes, the patient will know of another who underwent bariatric surgery; such persons can be vital sources of support in the postsurgical period. Another support system is of quite modern origin: There exist numerous online support groups, one of which may be of great use for the patient. Assuring the presence of a support system before surgery is a good means of ensuring long-term success.

P. Obstacles After Surgery

The interview usually ends with an exploration of potential obstacles after the surgery, many of which may have been suggested by the prior discussion. One must take into account the potential of spouses, family, work site, and community to create stress or postsurgical psychological barriers. These should be carefully analyzed, together with a discussion of what one should do to counter any obstacles that might develop.

Mostly often, patients will say, "I don't see any obstacles, everyone is behind me." They should then be told that surprises are not uncommon and should not be cause for undue dismay. If the patient has been hospitalized, this should be explored; although most have had positive experiences, this is not always true. In such cases, therapy may be important before the surgery to sort out any residual emotional issues.

Q. Summary

Some patients with morbid obesity have serious underlying psychological issues, which, if present, require professional attention prior to bariatric surgery. By combining standardized assessment tools with a structured interview, a psychologist can ensure that such problems are not present and better enable bariatric surgery to be successful.

R. Selected References

Chau WY, Schmidt HJ, Kouli W, et al. Patient characteristics impacting excess weight loss following laparoscopic adjustable gastric banding. Obes Surg 2005;15(3):346–350.

Choban PS, Onyejekwe J, Burge JC, et al. A health status assessment of the impact of weight loss following Roux-en-Y gastric bypass for clinically severe obesity. J Am Coll Surg 1999;188(5):491–497.

Frezza EE, Shebani KO, Wachtel MS. Laparoscopic gastric bypass for morbid obesity decreases bodily pain, improves physical functioning, and mental and general health in women. JLAST 2007;17(4):440–444.

Karl JG. Morbid obesity and related health risks. Ann Intern Med 1985;103:1043–1047.

Klesges RC, Klem M, Hansson CL. The effects of applicant's health status and qualifications on simulated hiring decisions. Int J Obesity 1990;14:527–535.

Kushner RF. Body weight and mortality. Nutr Rev 1993;51:127–136.

Naslund II, Agren G. Social and economic effects of bariatric surgery. Obes Surg 1991;1: 137–140.

Pagano M, Gauvreau K. Principles of biostatistics, 2nd ed. Pacific Grove, CA: Duxbury Thomson Learning, 2000.

Tarlov AR, Ware JE, Greenfield S, et al. An application of methods for monitoring the results of medical care. JAMA 1989;262:925–930.

Wadden TA, Stukard AJ. Social and psychological consequences of obesity. Ann Int Med 1985;103:1002–1012.

Ware JE, Sherbourne CD. The MOS 36-SF health Survey (SF 36). Concept framework and item selection. Med Care 1992;30:473–483.

www.parinc.com

www.wpspublish.com

8. Preoperative Check List

Rami R. Zanoun and Giselle G. Hamad

A. Introduction

The primary objectives of bariatric surgery are to improve obesity-related comorbidities and quality of life. The success of the bariatric surgical procedure relies not only on the technical expertise of the surgeon, but also on the proper preoperative evaluation and management of the patient's comorbid conditions.

In the preoperative setting, the bariatric surgeon should utilize a multidisciplinary approach for assessment and optimization of the various weight-related comorbidities of the bariatric patient. Once diagnostic studies have been reviewed, the surgeon can properly determine the patient's candidacy for surgery, assess the patient's surgical risk, and take preventive measures to minimize morbidity and mortality.

In addition to patient education, nutritional assessment, and evaluation of routine preoperative studies, a bariatric surgeon may recommend psychiatric and medical subspecialty consultation. Although the preoperative checklist serves as a reference guide for bariatric surgeons, each patient's case is unique and may require additional diagnostic studies.

The process of patient selection for bariatric surgery is unique for each surgeon because of the variation in a surgeon's bariatric surgical experience, personnel, hospital resources, and support.

B. Preoperative Testing

The goals of the preoperative testing are to assess the bariatric patient's operative risk and diagnose previously undiagnosed conditions. Table 8.1 lists routine laboratory tests and their corresponding indications. Additional testing may be indicated based on the patient's history and physical findings.

C. Preoperative Evaluation

1. Contraindications for bariatric surgery

Many clinicians regard the following conditions as absolute contraindications for performing bariatric surgery:

Table 8.1. Recommended preoperative testing.

Test	Indication
Complete blood count and platelet count	Routine preoperative bariatric laboratory evaluation
Basic metabolic panel, serum glucose	
Comprehensive metabolic panel, liver function tests	
Hemoglobin A1C	
Albumin	
TSH	
Fasting lipid panel/cholesterol	
Vitamin B$_{12}$, folate, thiamine levels	Exclude vitamin deficiency
Iron level	Exclude iron deficiency
Hypercoagulability testing (lupus anticoagulant assay, prothrombin gene variant, antithrombin III activity, Protein C and S levels and activity, activated protein C resistance, MTHFR homocysteine level, Factor V Leiden	Personal or family history of venous thromboembolism or hypercoagulable disorder
Upper endoscopy	Symptoms or diagnosis of gastroesophageal reflux disease or peptic ulcer disease
Colonoscopy	Patients ≥50 years or ≥40 years with first-degree family member with colon cancer, or 10 yrs younger than affected relative, whichever is earlier
Electrocardiogram	Men ≥40 years, women ≥50 years, history of arrhythmia, or younger patients with known coronary artery disease, hypertension, hypercholesterolemia, or diabetes mellitus
Echocardiogram	Heart murmur, valvular heart disease, or history of fenfluramine use
Chest radiograph	Age ≥50 years, known or suspected cardiac or pulmonary disease
Cardiac stress test or dobutamine echocardiogram	Refer to American Heart Association guidelines
Polysomnography	Snoring or Epworth score ≥10
Urine pregnancy test	Women of childbearing age
Pap smear	Exclude cervical cancer
Mammogram	Women ≥40 years
PSA	Men ≥50 years

Abbreviations: MTHFR, methylenetetrahydrofolate reductase; PSA, prostate specific antigen; TSH, thyroid-stimulating hormone.

a. mental impairment that interferes with a patient's ability to weigh the risks and benefits of surgery
b. active neoplastic disease
c. cirrhosis with portal hypertension
d. unstable or incurable pre-existing comorbidities, including unstable coronary artery disease (CAD), uncontrolled severe obstructive sleep apnea (OSA) with pulmonary hypertension, AIDS, or an uncontrolled psychiatric condition
e. pregnancy
f. immobility (e.g., wheelchair- or scooter-dependence)
g. inability or unwillingness to comply with postoperative regimens, including vitamin and mineral supplementation, dietary changes, and follow-up
h. active substance abuse

Several studies have shown that age alone is not a contraindication for bariatric surgery. However, when advanced age is combined with other severe medical comorbidities, the risk of surgery may become prohibitive.

2. Risk assessment

The mortality risk of bariatric surgery varies from 0.24% to 1.2% in the literature. The Obesity Surgery Mortality Risk Score, developed by DeMaria et al., utilizes five patient characteristics to stratify perioperative mortality for bariatric surgery:

a. male gender
b. age greater than or equal to 45 years
c. BMI greater than or equal to $50 \, kg/m^2$
d. hypertension
e. risk of pulmonary embolism

Each variable is scored as 1 point. In a multicenter study involving more than 4,000 patients, having zero to one, two to three, or four to five risk factors corresponded to mortality rates of 0.37%, 1.21%, and 2.4%, respectively.

D. Preoperative Checklist

1. Patient education

Encourage patient attendance at a bariatric surgical information session that explains the details of the procedure(s), alternatives, risks, benefits, insurance requirements, postoperative regimen, and recovery.

2. Nutritional counseling

Meeting with a registered dietitian can facilitate preoperative weight loss and promote a patient's ability to comply with postoperative dietary modifications and vitamin supplementation. Furthermore, involving the patient's family members can assist the patient in committing to these changes in lifestyle.

3. Psychological/psychiatric consultation

Many centers for bariatric surgery require psychological/psychiatric clearance. The aims are to determine whether the patient has the cognitive capacity to weigh the risks and benefits of surgery, diagnose occult mental illnesses that might require intervention, and ascertain whether the patient's psychiatric conditions pose undue risk to patient compliance with the postoperative regimen.

4. Informed consent

Discuss the course and risks of bariatric surgery.

a. Early complications: conversion to laparotomy, bleeding, infection, venous thromboembolism, anastomotic leak, intestinal obstruction, possible need for reoperation or readmission, and death.
b. Late complications: intestinal obstruction, marginal ulceration, internal hernia, stomal stenosis, cholelithiasis, band slippage and erosion, port site complications, failure of weight loss, and weight regain.
c. Discuss hospital course, including ambulation, incentive spirometry, pain control, drains and catheters, radiographic studies, length of hospital stay, and recovery time.
d. Discuss postoperative regimen, including dietary requirements, fluid intake, vitamin and mineral supplementation, exercise, and follow-up visits.
e. Discuss outcomes after bariatric surgery, including health benefits, improvement in quality of life, reduction in mortality, keys to success, and causes of failure of weight loss or weight regain.

5. Management of comorbidities

In order to reduce postoperative morbidity, proper measures must be undertaken to stabilize comorbid conditions.

a. Cardiac: High risk with coronary artery disease will require postoperative cardiac monitoring and may benefit from β-blockers administered perioperatively and postoperatively
b. Pulmonary: Patients with obstructive sleep apnea (OSA) should be encouraged to use their prescribed continuous positive airway pressure (CPAP) or bilevel positive airway pressure (BiPAP) treatments during sleep prior to the bariatric procedures [1, 3].
c. Thromboprophylaxis: For patients at high risk for venothromboembolic events (VTEs) (e.g., prior VTE, hypercoagulable disorder, venous stasis disease, obesity hypoventilation syndrome, BMI ≥60), consider inferior vena cava filter placement and/or extended anticoagulation.
d. Endocrine: Because of the elevated risk of infection, diabetics should be counseled to control hyperglycemia aggressively. Endocrinologic consultation may be necessary.

e. Gastrointestinal: Patients with gastroesophageal reflux disease should undergo upper endoscopy and may require proton pump inhibitor therapy and/or treatment of *Helicobacter pylori*.

f. Cholelithiasis: Ursodiol therapy has been shown to reduce the incidence of cholelithiasis after bariatric surgery. Some surgeons advocate routine prophylactic cholecystectomy during the bariatric procedure, whereas others perform cholecystectomy selectively in patients with symptomatic cholelithiasis.

g. Substance abuse: Smoking cessation and abstinence from alcohol or drug abuse is critical for reducing postoperative morbidity and promoting compliance.

6. Medication management

a. Discuss medications to discontinue prior to surgery (nonsteroidal anti-inflammatory drugs and aspirin, oral contraceptives, insulin, diuretics, and oral hypoglycemics).

b. For patients on Coumadin, discontinue Coumadin and order preoperative heparin or low-molecular-weight heparin.

c. Steroid-dependent patients will need perioperative stress-dose steroids.

E. Intraoperative Considerations

1. Ensure facility readiness

a. Armless chairs for patients in the waiting areas and patient rooms provide convenience and comfort. The wheelchairs, gurneys, operating room table, patient beds, and toilets must be able to accommodate the weight of bariatric patient comfortably. A bariatric bed may be required for patients whose weight exceeds the capacity of the standard hospital bed.

b. Air mattress transfer devices may be useful for transferring the patient to and from the operating table. They may be placed on the gurney in the holding area prior to surgery.

c. The operating table must be able to handle frequent changes in positioning, especially reverse Trendelenburg. A padded footboard is placed under the patient's plantar surfaces and the ankles are taped so that they do not rotate when the patient is in reverse Trendelenburg.

2. Prepare operating room equipment

a. Trocars
b. Insufflator
c. Light source
d. Camera
e. Video monitors
f. Angled laparoscope
g. Liver retractor

h. Laparoscopic graspers
i. Laparoscopic scissors
j. Suction and irrigation device
k. Clip appliers
l. Electrocautery
m. Ultrasonic shears
n. Linear and/or circular laparoscopic staplers and cartridges
o. Laparoscopic suturing devices or needle drivers
p. Upper endoscope

3. Prior to surgery

a. Identify patient upon arrival to the operating room.
b. The patient should be secured to the table because of frequent changes in table positioning during bariatric surgery. Pressure points should be well padded to prevent potential neuropathies.
c. Administer preoperative intravenous antibiotic prophylaxis.
d. Administer preoperative thromboprophylaxis (sequential compression devices activated prior to the induction of anesthesia and/or pharmacologic agents).
e. Perform Foley catheterization.

F. Conclusion

A successful outcome after bariatric surgery depends on optimization of medical conditions, patient education, postoperative compliance, and support from the bariatric surgical team, family, friends, and coworkers. A multidisciplinary approach is of critical importance and thorough preoperative preparation is mandatory.

G. Selected References

Collazo-Clavell ML, Clark MM, McAlpine DE, et al. Assessment and preparation of patients for bariatric surgery. Mayo Clin Proc 2006;81(10 Suppl):S11–17.

DeMaria EJ, Carmody BJ. Perioperative management of special populations: obesity. Surg Clin North Am 2005; 85(6):1283–1289, xii.

DeMaria EJ, Portenier D, Wolfe L. Obesity surgery mortality risk score: proposal for a clinically useful score to predict mortality risk in patients undergoing gastric bypass. Surg Obes Relat Dis 2007;3(2):134–140.

Flancbaum L, Belsley S. Factors affecting morbidity and mortality of Roux-en-Y gastric bypass for clinically severe obesity: an analysis of 1,000 consecutive open cases by a single surgeon. J Gastrointest Surg 2007;11:500–507.

Hamad GG, Bergqvist D. Venous thromboembolism in bariatric surgery patients: an update of risk and prevention. Surg Obes Relat Dis 2007;3(1):97–102.

Kuruba R, Koche LS, Murr MM. Preoperative assessment and perioperative care of patients undergoing bariatric surgery. Med Clin North Am 2007;91(3):339–351, ix.

Mason EE, Renquist KE, Huang YH, et al. Causes of 30-day bariatric surgery mortality: with emphasis on bypass obstruction. Obes Surg 2007;17(1):9–14.

McGlinch BP, Que FG, Nelson JL, et al. Perioperative care of patients undergoing bariatric surgery. Mayo Clin Proc 2006;81(10 Suppl):S25–33.

Schirmer B, Erenoglu C, Miller A. Flexible endoscopy in the management of patients undergoing Roux-en-Y gastric bypass. Obes Surg 2002;12:634–638.

Sugerman HJ, Brewer WH, Shiffman ML, et al. A multicenter, placebo-controlled, randomized, double-blind, prospective trial of prophylactic ursodiol for the prevention of gallstone formation following gastric-bypass-induced rapid weight loss. Am J Surg 1995;169(1):91–96; discussion 96–97.

9. Postoperative Care Pathway

Daniel M. Herron and Murali N. Naidu

A. Rationale for Care Pathways

Bariatric patients, both because of their size and comorbid conditions, present many unique issues in their postoperative care. The utilization of postoperative care pathways can help to address these issues, provide a more uniformly high level of care, and minimize the risk of in-hospital postoperative complications. Furthermore, care pathways can reduce the variability in care that occurs due to changes in resident and nursing staff. Suggested postoperative orders for laparoscopic gastric bypass and laparoscopic adjustable gastric band patients are provided at the end of this chapter.

B. General Guidelines for Postoperative Hospitalization and Monitoring

1. Length of stay

The length of stay for bariatric patients is generally quite short. With this narrow window to identify potentially life-threatening postoperative complications, care guidelines regarding nursing care and patient monitoring are extremely helpful in identifying complications early.

    a. The typical laparoscopic gastric bypass patient spends two nights in the hospital. Some centers have reduced the stay to a single night.

    b. Laparoscopic adjustable gastric band patients are admitted for a single night, or may even be treated as outpatients.

    c. Duodenal switch patients follow a postoperative course similar to gastric bypass patients. However, they are substantially more likely to require additional days due to postoperative pain and nausea.

    d. Sleeve gastrectomy patients follow a postoperative course similar to gastric bypass patients.

2. Nursing care guidelines

    a. Bariatric patients with minimal comorbidities may be safely transferred from the recovery room directly to the floor.

    b. Patients with cardiac or pulmonary issues, particularly sleep apnea, may benefit from a monitored setting such as a stepdown unit. Routine use of the ICU is unnecessary, unless it is the only monitored setting available.

c. Vital signs should be checked at least every 4 hours and more frequently if possible.

d. Fever greater than 38.5 °C, tachycardia above 110, oliguria, a patient who "doesn't look right" or who describes a sense of "impending doom" should trigger a call to a physician for further evaluation. These findings may be the first indication that a leak is present and should not be ignored. The threshold for leak or sepsis workup must be very low.

e. It is critically important that all caregivers understand that physical exam of the abdomen in a morbidly obese patient is unreliable. The obese abdomen may appear benign on exam, even in the presence of florid peritonitis; this must be clear to all personnel involved in post-operative care so that an expedited workup for postoperative leak or sepsis may be initiated if needed.

C. Postoperative Tubes and Drains

1. Nasogastric tubes

Most surgeons performing laparoscopic bariatric procedures do not routinely leave a nasogastric tube in after surgery. While these tubes may be inserted during the operation to decompress the stomach or check for leaks, they are typically removed in the operating room. If a nasogastric tube is left after an open bariatric procedure, it may usually be removed on the first postoperative day. Nasogastric tubes generally should not be reinserted after removal.

2. Intra-abdominal drains

Data regarding the routine use of intra-abdominal drains are controversial, but most surgeons feel that their use does not improve outcome. If drains are used, they should be left in place until the time of greatest risk of leakage has passed, generally 2 to 7 days after surgery.

3. Foley catheters

A urinary catheter may be placed during surgery and left in postoperatively. In addition to providing an accurate measurement of the patient's urine output, it may contribute to the patient's comfort.

D. Deep Vein Thrombosis Prophylaxis

Since deep vein thrombosis with pulmonary embolism is one of the most feared and potentially lethal complications of bariatric surgery, all bariatric patients should receive at least one form of prophylaxis. At present, there is no general consensus regarding the best protocol.

1. Sequential compression devices

Most institutions use sequential compression devices starting before the induction of anesthesia and continuing until the patient is fully ambulatory or discharged.

2. Heparin therapy

Bariatric patients are generally given nonfractionated heparin 5,000 units subcutaneously every 8 hours.

a. Note the more frequent dosing of nonfractionated heparin in the morbidly obese population compared with the twice-daily dosage used in the nonobese.

b. Heparin therapy may be started before the surgical procedure or immediately thereafter. Some surgeons feel that its use before surgery may increase the risk of bleeding in the early postoperative period, although this has not been confirmed.

c. Fractionated heparin may also be used.

E. Use of Bariatric Beds

Hospital beds are gradually being manufactured in larger sizes as our population continues to grow heavier. Typical hospital beds will accommodate patients up to 350 lbs or 28 in. wide without difficulty. Heavier or wider patients require specially designed bariatric beds. In addition to stronger construction, these beds often provide the ability to take on a chair configuration and assist the patient in getting OOB to a standing position.

F. Postoperative Diet

1. General dietary guidelines

Most bariatric programs utilize special dietary regimens for their patients; these are often given special names such as "Stage I," "Stage II," etc. to differentiate them from nonbariatric diets.

a. In general, bariatric diets consist of small portions of low-calorie, low-sugar, low-fat items.

b. The use of small "shot-glass" size cups will remind patients to drink small amounts.

c. Carbonated beverages and caffeine are avoided in the early postoperative phase. Some surgeons tell their patients to permanently avoid carbonation on the theory that it may stretch the gastric pouch.

d. Concentrated sweets should be avoided as these may trigger dumping syndrome in the gastric bypass patient. Standard general surgical postoperative diets such as the traditional "clear liquid diet" may contain substantial amounts of carbohydrate and should be avoided.

2. Postoperative diet progression

Every program has a unique approach to dietary advancement. It is important that patients are educated in advance regarding their particular program's approach. We have found that it is helpful to provide patients with a handout delineating the dietary progression well in advance of their operation. This allows the patient to purchase foods and drinks before admission so that they are available after discharge. Nurses, nutritional staff, and ancillary personnel should be educated regarding the special dietary needs of the postbariatric patient.

   a. Liquids (Stage I)
       The first diet consists of sips of low-calorie, noncarbonated liquids. Noncaloric sweeteners may be used. This diet may be given to laparoscopic gastric bypass patients on their first postoperative day, or to adjustable gastric band patients immediately following surgery.
   b. Pureed (Stage II)
       Some programs maintain patients on a liquid diet during their entire inpatient stay. Others advance them to a pureed diet as soon as the second postoperative day. The Stage II diet is also low-calorie, low-fat, and without carbonated beverages.
   c. Solid (Stage III)
       Most surgeons wait until the stomach is fully healed (3–4 weeks) before finally advancing their patients to solid food.

2. Vitamins, minerals, and medications

   a. Most surgeons start patients on supplementation postoperatively. Multivitamins or calcium should be chewable or liquid during the early postoperative phase.
   b. Iron supplementation should be avoided in the early postoperative phase, as it may exacerbate constipation while the patient is still taking narcotic pain medication.

3. Oral medications

Most patients tolerate oral medication adequately, even during the immediate postoperative phase, although very large pills may need to be cut in pieces or crushed, if possible.

G. Postoperative Imaging

1. Routine upper GI series

   a. Gastric bypass
       Routine postoperative imaging has not been shown to reduce morbidity or mortality after laparoscopic gastric bypass surgery. However, many surgeons believe that obtaining such imaging in the early stages of a new bariatric program will generate expertise among the radiology

and surgery staff by providing knowledge of normal postoperative anatomy.

b. Adjustable gastric band

Routine upper GI series is useful after laparoscopic adjustable gastric band placement. It provides a baseline indication of band positioning that will prove valuable in the future if there is concern about prolapse or slippage. It also confirms patency of the band, which guides diet advancement.

2. Selective imaging workup

a. Upper GI series

This study is very useful in evaluating the febrile, tachycardic, or oliguric patient, or even the patient who "just doesn't look right." The upper GI series (UGI) is considered to be the gold standard for demonstrating leaks from the gastric pouch or proximal anastomosis, but is ineffective in evaluating the distal anastomosis. If a leak is suspected distal to the gastrojejunostomy, immediate return to the operating room should be considered.

b. Computed tomography scan

Computed tomography (CT) is useful in evaluating the gastric pouch, proximal anastomosis and distal anastomosis. It should be remembered that CO_2 insufflation is generally resorbed by 24 hours and that free intra-abdominal gas seen after that time should raise the suspicion of a leak.

c. The negative study

UGI and CT are not 100% sensitive! A negative imaging study should never preclude a return to the operating room if there is suspicion of an intra-abdominal leak.

3. Choice of contrast

Water-soluble contrast such as Gastrografin should be used in the early postoperative period, although barium is also safe if the possibility of a leak has been ruled out.

H. Pain Management

In general, patients have less postoperative pain after a laparoscopic procedure than an open one. Nonetheless, it remains important to ensure that even laparoscopic patients have access to adequate postoperative pain control. Some bariatric programs use a combination of scheduled parenteral nonsteroidal anti-inflammatory drugs (NSAIDs; e.g., ketorolac) in conjunction with an injectable narcotic as needed. Others find that patient-controlled analgesia (PCA) plays a valuable role in postoperative pain control. Aggressive control of postoperative pain aids in early ambulation, which improves pulmonary mechanics and reduces the risk of DVT/PE. Use of NSAIDs should be immediately discontinued if there is suspicion of postoperative bleeding.

I. Postoperative Antibiotics

We routinely provide a weight-adjusted dose of first-generation cephalosporin 30 minutes prior to incision. As with other clean-contaminated cases, there is no Level I evidence supporting prophylactic postoperative antibiotics.

J. Consolidation of Postoperative Ordersets in Bariatric Postoperative Ordersets

Every effort should be made to formalize the bariatric management concepts described here into a written care protocol that includes printed or computerized ordersets and formal nursing care pathways. Without such formal organization, it is inevitable that important components such as DVT prophylaxis will be sporadically missed. While postoperative care protocols do not guarantee a good outcome, their use increases compliance and optimizes care. Sample ordersets for laparoscopic gastric bypass and laparoscopic adjustable gastric banding are given in the following.

Appendix I. Sample Postlaparoscopic Gastric Bypass Orderset

(Please note that these sample ordersets serve as a framework only; they should not be copied word-for-word and must be individualized for each patient and hospital.)

Postoperative orders

- Admit patient to recovery; transfer to stepdown unit if sleep apnea present; otherwise transfer to floor when stable
- Use bariatric bed if patient weighs over 350 lbs
- Diagnosis: S/P laparoscopic gastric bypass
- Condition: Stable
- Vital signs q 2 hours for 12 hours, then q 4 hours
- OOB with assistance starting today
- Sequential compression device to both legs while in bed
- Record strict I/Os
- Foley catheter to gravity bag
- Incentive spirometry per routine
- Notify MD for T > 38.4 °C, HR > 110, Systolic BP < 100
- NPO except ice chips and medications with a sip of water
- IV: D5LR @ 150 cc/hour
- Heparin 5,000 Units SubQ q8 hours
- Ketorolac 30 mg IV q6 hours

- Hydromorphone 2–4 mg IV prn breakthrough pain
- Ondansetron 4 mg IV q6 hours PRN nausea/vomiting
- Labs: CBC in AM tomorrow
- (Remember to resume cardiac medications and CPAP if required, and monitor glucose appropriately for diabetic patients.)

Postoperative day #1

- If T > 38.4 °C or HR > 110, Upper GI series with Gastrografin to rule out leak
- Notify MD immediately if study is positive
- If study was not needed or is negative:
  - Remove Foley catheter
  - Advance diet to Bariatric Stage I (low calorie, noncarbonated liquids, small portions)
  - Heplock IV when tolerating diet
  - Out of bed and ambulate with assistance at least TID

Postoperative day #2

- Advance diet to Bariatric Stage II (low-calorie pureed, small portion)
- Discontinue hydromorphone
- Acetaminophen/oxycodone 325/5 mg 1–2 tabs po q 4 hrs PRN pain; take crushed with yogurt or applesauce
- Review all discharge teaching with patient; give printed instructions
- Discharge home when tolerating Stage II diet and pain well controlled

Appendix II. Sample postlaparoscopic adjustable gastric band orderset

(Please note that these sample ordersets serve as a framework only; they should not be copied word-for-word and must be individualized for each patient and hospital.)

Postoperative orders

- Admit patient to recovery; transfer to stepdown unit if sleep apnea present; otherwise, transfer to floor when stable
- Use bariatric bed if patient weighs over 350 lbs
- Diagnosis: S/P laparoscopic adjustable gastric band
- Condition: Stable
- Vital signs q 2 hours for 12 hours, then q 4 hours
- OOB with assistance starting today
- Sequential compression device to both legs while in bed
- Record strict I/Os
- Foley catheter to gravity bag

- Incentive spirometry per routine
- Notify MD for T > 38.4 °C, HR > 110, Systolic BP < 100
- Diet: Bariatric Stage I (low calorie, noncarbonated liquids, small portions)
- IV: D5LR @ 150 cc/hour
- Heparin 5,000 Units SC q8 hours
- Ketorolac 30 mg IV q6 hours
- Hydromorphone 2–4 mg IV prn breakthrough pain
- Ondansetron 4 mg IV q6 hours PRN nausea/vomiting
- Labs: CBC in AM tomorrow
- Schedule Gastrografin swallow for tomorrow AM
- (Remember to resume cardiac medications and CPAP if required, and monitor glucose appropriately for diabetic patients.)

Postoperative day #1

- IF UGI shows leak or malpositioned band, contact MD immediately.
- If UGI study is negative for leak and band is in good position:

  o Remove Foley catheter.
  o Advance diet to Bariatric Stage II (low calorie pureed, small portions).
  o Heplock IV when tolerating diet.
  o Out of bed and ambulate with assistance at least TID.
  o Discontinue hydromorphone.
  o Acetaminophen/Hydromorphone 325/5 mg 1–2 tabs po q 4 hrs PRN pain; take crushed with yogurt or applesauce.
  o Review all discharge teaching with patient; give printed instructions.
  o Discharge home when tolerating Stage II diet and pain well controlled.

Selected References

Cooney RN, Bryant P, Haluck R, et al. The impact of a clinical pathway for gastric bypass surgery on resource utilization. J Surg Res 2001;98:97–101.

Herron DM. The surgical management of severe obesity. Mt Sinai J Med 2004;71:63–71.

Herron DM. Establishing and organizing a bariatric surgery program. In: Inabnet WB, DeMaria EJ, Ikramuddin S, eds. Laparoscopic bariatric surgery. Philadelphia: Lippincott Williams & Wilkins, 2005.

Huerta S, Heber D, Sawicki MP, et al. Reduced length of stay by implementation of a clinical pathway for bariatric surgery in an academic health care center. Am Surg 2001;67:1128–1135.

Pieracci FM, Barie PS, Pomp A. Critical care of the bariatric patient. Crit Care Med 2006;34:1796–1804.

Yeats M, Wedergren S, Fox N, et al. The use and modification of clinical pathways to achieve specific outcomes in bariatric surgery. Am Surg 2005;71:152–154.

10. Long-term Follow-up Protocol of Bariatric Patients

Steven Teich and Marc P. Michalsky

A. Introduction

Bariatric procedures induce weight loss using a combination of restrictive and/or malabsorptive surgical techniques. The metabolic and nutritional complications of bariatric surgery are, in part, directly related to the surgically created anatomical changes in the gastrointestinal tract. They also occur due to patient noncompliance with nutritional supplementation and dietary alterations following surgery. Despite having huge stores of energy in the form of excess fat, morbidly obese patients (BMI $\geq 35\,kg/m^2$) may have clinical or subclinical nutritional deficiencies preoperatively as a consequence of poor diet over a prolonged period of time. Therefore, the severity of the postoperative nutritional deficit is dependent on several factors, including the patient's preoperative nutritional status, the specific bariatric procedure undertaken, postoperative complications, patient-related nutritional compliance, and routine follow-up with his or her surgeon and primary care provider.

At the end of this chapter we have included Tables 10.1 to 10.3, which describe the site of absorption of nutrients, mechanism of action of various bariatric surgical procedures, and common nutritional and metabolic complications of bariatric surgery. Table 10.4 contains suggested mineral and vitamin supplementation following various bariatric surgical procedures, and Table 10.5 provides recommended screening tests prior to bariatric surgery and postoperatively.

B. Vitamin Deficiencies

1. Vitamin B_{12} and folate

Vitamin B_{12} deficiency is common after bariatric surgery when restrictive procedures such as Roux-en-Y gastric bypass (RYGB) are utilized. The parietal cells that secrete acid and intrinsic factor and the chief cells that secrete pepsinogen are mainly located in the fundus and body of the stomach. The small residual pouch created with the RYGB has minimal acid production and pepsin-related digestion of protein-bound cobalamins in food. This coupled with decreased production of intrinsic factor means that vitamin B_{12} cannot be separated from foods and crystalline B_{12} cannot be absorbed in the terminal ileum. The prevalence of B_{12} deficiency after RYGB is 12% to 33%, but clinical symptoms are less prevalent. The body storage of vitamin B_{12} is large compared to daily needs;

the normal human reserve is 2 to 5 years. Therefore, vitamin B_{12} deficiency can appear years after surgery; so patients undergoing RYGB need to be monitored long-term and treated with vitamin B_{12} once they demonstrate low blood levels. The most common clinical manifestations of B_{12} deficiency are macrocytic anemia and neurologic symptoms (i.e., peripheral neuropathy, paresthesias, and demyelination of the corticospinal and dorsal columns).

Folate deficiency, while less frequent than B_{12} deficiency, occurs mainly due to reduced dietary intake but also occurs secondary to reduced gastric acid and lack of exposure to the upper small intestine. Folate is absorbed primarily from the proximal third of the small intestine, but with adaptation it can be absorbed along the entire length of the small bowel. Folate deficiency occurs in 9-35% of bypass patients and presents as megaloblastic anemia. It is promptly corrected with multivitamin supplementation (1 mg folate/day).

2. Thiamine

Thiamine is normally absorbed in the acid environment of the duodenum. Thiamine deficiency occurs through reduced acid production by the gastric pouch, reduced dietary intake, and frequent vomiting. Severe thiamine deficiency leads to Wernicke encephalopathy, which consists of ocular changes (nystagmus and ocular nerve palsies), ataxia, and apathetic mental confusion. Acute thiamine deficiency requires parental thiamine 50 to 200 mg per day until symptoms resolve, then 50 to 100 mg daily by mouth. However, thiamine deficiency can usually be prevented with a daily multivitamin.

3. Calcium and vitamin D

Calcium deficiency after RYGB and biliopancreatic diversion (BPD) is common due to the surgically induced changes. Reduced calcium absorption occurs secondary to exclusion of the duodenum and proximal jejunum, where maximal calcium absorption occurs. Vitamin D is preferentially absorbed in the jejunum and ileum. Calcium malabsorption is aggravated by the defective absorption of fat and fat-soluble vitamins, including vitamin D. The lack of calcium results in increased production of parathormone (PTH), which then causes increased production of 1,25 dihydroxy-vitamin D and increased release of calcium from bone. Slater et al. found that over the first 4 years post-BPD the incidence of hypocalcemia increased from 15% to 48%, with a corresponding increase in PTH levels in 69% of patients.

Monitoring for calcium deficiency must include serum calcium, ionized calcium, serum phosphorus, alkaline phosphatase, PTH, and 25(OH) vitamin D levels. All patients undergoing RYGB and BPD require a high intake of calcium (2 g/day) along with calcium supplementation (1,200–1,500 mg elemental calcium/day) and vitamin D (400 IU/day). Calcium citrate rather than calcium carbonate should be prescribed because it is more soluble in the absence of stomach acid.

4. Vitamin A

Vitamin A, along with the other fat-soluble vitamins D, E, and K, diffuse across the brush border plasma membrane of the intestinal epithelial cell inside micelles formed by bile salts and lipids. The majority of fat-soluble vitamin absorption occurs in the proximal two thirds of the jejunum. Deficiencies occur following malabsorptive procedures due to bypassing the duodenum and a variable length of jejunum with inadequate mixing of food with biliary and pancreatic secretions, causing steatorrhea, bile salt wasting, and malabsorption of fat soluble vitamins. Vitamin A deficiency is associated with eye disease: night blindness, xerophthalmia, Bitot's spots, and keratomalacia. Skin manifestations of vitamin A deficiency include xerosis and petechiae. The current recommendation for vitamin A replacement therapy is 25,000 IU daily.

C. Mineral Deficiencies

1. Iron

Iron deficiency and anemia occur frequently in preoperative as well as postoperative bariatric patients. The postoperative causes of iron deficiency include decreased absorption of iron due to bypass of the duodenum, decreased gastric acid (which is needed to reduce iron to its more absorbable ferrous form), and reduced iron intake from avoidance of certain foods. Symptoms of iron deficiency include fatigue, glossitis, stomatitis, and complaints of feeling cold due to impaired temperature regulation. The incidence of preoperative iron deficiency is reported to be between 14% and 44%. Postoperative iron deficiency occurs in 20% to 74% of patients undergoing RYGB, with the greatest risk in menstruating women. All patients undergoing bariatric surgery should receive supplementation, but noncompliance is a problem due to gastrointestinal intolerance and constipation.

There are many iron supplementation regimens with various forms of iron therapy. Some examples include iron gluconate or sulfate 40 to 65 mg three times per day and ferrous sulfate 320 mg twice per day. Adding vitamin C to iron therapy is beneficial because it promotes iron absorption. The amount of iron supplementation should be increased if iron deficiency anemia is present or if the hemoglobin level falls below 11 g/dl.

2. Zinc

Zinc deficiency causes hair loss, dermatitis, impaired immunity, and delayed wound healing. In the postoperative bariatric patient it can be due to bypass of the primary site of zinc absorption in the small intestine, reduced intake of foods that provide zinc, and increased stool losses due to steatorrhea. In patients who have normal zinc levels preoperatively, zinc supplementation should be initiated within 2 months after bariatric surgery. Zinc intake as well as serum and urinary levels should be followed after surgery.

3. Copper

Copper is essential to the structure and function of the nervous system. In postoperative bariatric patients copper deficiency can present as a neuropathy of the lower extremities. Copper is likely absorbed in the stomach and duodenum. When prescribing high-dose zinc supplementation it is important to recognize that copper absorption is inhibited due to increasing levels of copper-binding protein.

D. Selected References

Brolin RE. Gastric bypass. Surg Clin North Am 2001;81:1077–1095.

Brolin RE, Gorman JH, Gorman RC, et al. Prophylactic iron supplementation after Roux-en-Y gastric bypass: a prospective, double-blind, randomized study. Arch Surg 1998;133:740–744.

Brolin RE, Leung M. Survey of vitamin and mineral supplementation after gastric bypass and biliopancreatic diversion for morbid obesity. Obes Surg 1999;9:150–154.

Carrodeguas L, Kaidar-Person O, Szomstein S, et al. Preoperative thiamine deficiency in obese population undergoing laparoscopic bariatric surgery. Surg Obes Relat Dis 2005;1:517–522.

Cominetti C, Garrido AB Jr, Cozzolino SM. Zinc nutritional status of morbidly obese patients before and after Roux-en-Y gastric bypass: a preliminary report. Obes Surg 2006;16:448–453.

Flancbaum L, Belsley S, Drake V, et al. Preoperative nutritional status of patients undergoing Roux-en-Y gastric bypass for morbid obesity. J Gastrointest Surg 2006;10:1033–1037.

Goldenberg L. Nutritional deficiencies following bariatric surgery. Obesity Care Special Edition. 2007;Summer 65–72.

Kalfarentzos F, Kechagias I, Soulikia K, et al. Weight loss following vertical banded gastroplasty: intermediate results of a prospective study. Obes Surg 2001;11:265–270.

Kumar N, Ahlskog JE, Gross JB. Acquired hypocupremia after gastric surgery. Clin Gastroenterol Hepatol 204;2:1074–1079.

Kushner R. Managing micronutrient deficiencies in the bariatric surgical patient. Obesity Mgmt 2005;203–206.

Madan AK, Orth WS, Tichansky DS, et al. Vitamin and trace mineral levels after laparoscopic gastric bypass. Obes Surg 2006;16:603–606.

Malinowski SS. Nutritional and metabolic complications of bariatric surgery. Am J Med Sci 2006;4:219–225.

Rhode BM, Shustik C, Christou NV, et al. Iron absorption and therapy after gastric bypass. Obes Surg 1999;9:17–21.

Sheu WH, Wu HS, Wang CV, et al. Elevated plasma homocysteine concentrations six months after gastroplasty in morbidly obese subjects. Intern Med 2001;40:584–588.

Skroubis G, Sakellaropoulos G, Pouggouras K, et al. Comparison of nutritional deficiencies after Roux-en-Y gastric bypass. Obes Surg 2002;12:551–558.

Slater GH, Ren CJ, Siegel N, et al. Serum fat-soluble vitamin deficiency and abnormal calcium metabolism after malabsorptive bariatric surgery. J Gastrointest Surg 2004;8:48–55.

Tucker ON, Szomstein S, Rosenthal RJ. Nutritional consequences of weight-loss surgery. Med Clin North Am 2007;499–514.

Table 10.1. Site of absorption of nutrients.

Intestinal site of absorption	Nutrients
Duodenum	Calcium
	Thiamine
	Iron
	Protein
	Carbohydrate
Jejunum/proximal ileum	Fat
	Vitamins A, D, E, K
	Water-soluble vitamins
	Folate
	Essential minerals
	Copper
	Zinc
	Phosphorus
	Magnesium
Terminal ileum	Vitamin B_{12}
	Bile salts

Table 10.2. Mechanism of action of surgical procedures.

Surgical procedure	Mechanism of action
Roux-en-Y gastric bypass	1[ary] restriction/2[ary] malabsorption
Adjustable gastric band	Purely restriction
Sleeve gastrectomy	Purely restriction
Biliopancreatic diversion	1[ary] malabsorption/2[ary] restriction

Table 10.3. Common nutritional and metabolic complications of bariatric procedures.

Roux-en-Y gastric bypass	Biliopancreatic diversion
Vitamin B_{12} deficiency	Vitamin B_{12} deficiency
Iron deficiency	Iron deficiency
Thiamine deficiency	Folate deficiency
Metabolic bone disease	Thiamine deficiency
Cholelithiasis	Fat-soluble vitamin deficiency
	Calcium deficiency
	Metabolic bone disease
	Cholelithiasis
	Fat malabsorption
	Severe malnutrition

Table 10.4. Suggested mineral and vitamin supplementation following bariatric surgery.

Roux-en-Y gastric bypass	Laparoscopic adjustable gastric band	Sleeve gastrectomy	Biliopancreatic diversion
Multivitamin tablet with minerals (1 tablet/day)	Multivitamin tablet with minerals (1 tablet/day)	Multivitamin tablet with minerals (1 tablet/day)	Multivitamin tablet with minerals (1 tablet/day)
Vitamin A 1 mg/day	Vitamin A 1 mg/day	Vitamin A 1 mg/day	Vitamin A 1 mg/day
Vitamin D 5 mcg/day	Vitamin D 5 μg/day	Vitamin D 5 μg/day	Vitamin D 5 μg/day
Vitamin E 100–300 mg/day	Vitamin E 100–300 mg/day	Vitamin E 100–300 mg/day	Vitamin E 100–300 mg/day
Vitamin K 65–80 μg/day	Vitamin K 65–80 μg/day	Vitamin K 65–80 μg/day	Vitamin K 65–80 μg/day
Vitamin B_{12} (350–500 μg/day) daily-oral (100-300 μg/day) or sublingual (500 μg/day) monthly-IM (1,000 μg/day)		Vitamin B_{12} (350–500 μg/day) daily-oral (100–300 μg/day) or sublingual (500 μg/day)	Vitamin B_{12} (350–500 μg/day) daily-oral (100–300 μg/day) or sublingual (500 μg/day) monthly-IM (1,000 μg/day)
Vitamin B complex with thiamine (1 tablet/day)	Vitamin B complex with thiamine (1 tablet/day)	Vitamin B complex with thiamine (1 tablet/day)	Vitamin B complex with thiamine (1 tablet/day)
Calcium citrate or calcium lactate with vitamin D (1,200–1,500 mg/day)	Calcium citrate or calcium lactate with vitamin D (1,200–1,500 mg/day)	Calcium citrate or calcium lactate with vitamin D (1,200–1,500 mg/day)	Calcium citrate or calcium lactate with vitamin D (1,200–1,500 mg/day)
Ferrous sulfate or gluconate (325–650 mg/day) (increase in menstruating women)	Ferrous sulfate or gluconate (325–650 mg/day) (increase in menstruating women)	Ferrous sulfate or gluconate (325–650 mg/day) (increase in menstruating women)	Ferrous sulfate or gluconate (325–650 mg/day) (increase in menstruating women)
Vitamin C (500 mg/day)	Vitamin C (500 mg/day)	Vitamin C (500 mg/day)	Vitamin C (500 mg/day)
Zinc (15 mg/day)	Zinc (15 mg/day)	Zinc (15 mg/day)	Zinc (15 mg/day)
Biotin (3,000 μg/day)	Biotin (3,000 μg/day)	Biotin (3,000 μg/day)	Biotin (3,000 μg/day)

Source: Data from Malinowski SS (2006), Goldenberg L (2007), and Tucker ON et al. (2007).

Table 10.5. Recommended screening tests prior to bariatric surgery and postoperatively (3 months, 6 months, 1 year, then annually).

CBC, PT/PTT
Lipid profile
Hg A_{1c}
Iron studies: Serum iron, TIBC, ferritin, transferrin
Serum folate and vitamin B_{12}
Thiamine (vitamin B_1)
Serum albumin and prealbumin
Serum chemistries: including calcium, magnesium, and phosphorus
Vitamin A
Vitamin D_{25}—total
Selenium, zinc, ceruloplasmin (copper)
PTH

Source: Data from Goldenberg L (2007) and Tucker ON et al. (2007).

11. An Economic Approach to Opening a Bariatric Practice

Bradley T. Ewing and Eldo E. Frezza

A. Introduction

Nearly one fourth of all Americans are obese or morbidly obese. In fact, the number of morbidly obese persons has been increasing over time and this trend is expected to continue. Not surprisingly, many physicians are considering specializing in bariatrics and opening new practices.

From a business standpoint, the decision to open a bariatric practice should be based on whether or not the enterprise can achieve an acceptable rate of profit. The application of economic tools in conjunction with techniques of operations management can increase the likelihood that this decision will be optimal. Clearly, the central question of whether to take on a project such as opening a specialized practice is: Do the benefits outweigh the costs? The guidelines presented here focus on identifying factors that lead to value enhancement; the bariatric physician should consider these when making decisions about the business side of his or her practice.

B. Outline the Business

Prior to opening a practice, it is necessary for the bariatric physician to outline the business and operations strategy, mission statement, core competencies, and service and process design for the bariatric services to be provided. This overall plan has several purposes. First, this plan is geared at providing a market forecast of the service provision (i.e., production) requirements for the future. Secondly, this plan deals with analyzing and selecting a service location or locations, and planning the capacity of the practice facility. Additionally, this plan is designed to provide information on what the practice facility will look like and how it will function. Our approach to the business model of opening a bariatric practice relies on sound economic principles, knowledge of operations management and business strategy, as well as a fundamental understanding of bariatric medicine.

C. Mission Statement

As is true of any successful business venture, a company must know who or what it is. In order to position itself for the future, that is, to be able to make profit in both good times and bad, a strong sense of mission is required. Thus, the first step in our model is to create a mission statement. The mission statement clearly and concisely answers three questions:

1. What business is our practice *really* in?
2. Who will be the customers?
3. How will the practice's basic beliefs define the business?

Key components of mission and vision statements include brief descriptions of the business, customers, and core competencies. For example, will the practice be in the business of providing healthy and sustainable lifestyle changes or simply weight loss solutions? Notice how the former suggests ongoing care for patients and allows for future technologies and advances in medicine to define the specific procedures that the practice may provide. The latter, weight loss solutions, is narrowly defined and may not fully capture plans for follow-up care, recurrence, and other issues such as preventive medical services.

The customers of the practice may be the patients themselves (narrow view) or extend to family members of those affected by bariatric patients (broader view) to society in general (broadest view). The choice of customer market focus is important and will guide the type of services, doctors and nurses, procedures, location, and even purchases of equipment that your practice will acquire and utilize.

Core competencies are those things that a company does better than everyone else. They are those activities or abilities that should be focused on no matter what is currently happening in the industry or economy. For example, if a practice provides personal attention better than anything else, then it will be optimal for decisions to be made with this in mind. The practice will do best by asking, "Is this activity (purchase, new service, etc.) in line with our core competencies?" If it is not, then it is often the case that the activity under question will be a drag on resources. A rule of thumb is that the core competencies will align well with the values and belief systems of the organization. A mission statement that is clear from the onset is capable of guiding decision making far into the future and thus defining the economic scope and scale of the practice for years to come.

D. Competitive Advantages and Priorities

How does a practice gain a competitive advantage in the market place? The answer to this question comes from the practice's core competencies. In order to take full advantage of core competencies, it is necessary to determine one's competitive priorities. There are four broad categories of competitive priorities: cost, quality, time (speed), and flexibility. It is crucial to determine on which of these the new practice will concentrate most. It is here where the practice can differentiate itself from others. Firms that compete on:

*   *Cost* are the low-cost provider.
*   *Quality* offer the "best" service.
*   *Time (speed)* offer services in the most timely manner.
*   *Flexibility* are able to change or alter their mix of services quickly.

Each of these priorities is an admirable goal and many firms excel by focusing on all of them to some extent. However, economic trade-offs are often involved in choosing one priority over another; therefore, a balance must be struck. For example, it is difficult to offer the highest quality service (since it is costly for the provider) and simultaneously offer the services at the lowest cost to patients. Successful businesses tend to choose one priority that will be the basis for competing in the marketplace while maintaining a desired level or standard for the other priorities. Thus, a practice may choose a quality level (e.g., private rooms or semiprivate rooms) and then, for that level of quality, provide the services at the lowest cost to patients.

Overall, the business strategy of the practice comes from these competitive priorities. The key to success and the optimal operation of the practice is to know how they will support the corporate strategy or mission of the practice.

E. Environmental Scanning

Understanding the economic environment in which the practice will operate is critical for making good decisions. The focus of environmental scanning is on identifying market trends, opportunities, existing strengths, and threats or weaknesses. A standard tool for this portion of the business planning model is the strengths, weaknesses, opportunities, and threats (SWOT) analysis. A general framework for the SWOT analysis is as follows:

1. Identify generic issues or problem areas: ethics, leadership, facilities, planning, political, technology, legal, etc.
2. Develop a list of facts pertaining to the issues or problem areas.
3. Determine whether each fact is *internal* (i.e., practice has the power to change or influence this issue or problem) or *external* to the practice.
4. Value the factoids from on a scale from weak (−10) to strong (+10), with 0 being neutral.
5. Limit the compiled list to those items valued at either −10 or +10.

The results of the SWOT analysis can be interpreted based on the following:

- Strengths: facts with high, positive, internal values
- Weaknesses: facts with high, negative, internal values
- Opportunities: facts with high, positive, external values
- Threats: facts with high, negative, external values

Knowledge gained from a SWOT analysis allows the firm to develop strategies to overcome potential problems as well as how to exploit existing strengths and opportunities.

Other methods of assessing the economic environment include economic impact analysis (EIA) at the regional, state and national levels. Obesity and its associated illnesses are known to lower productivity and wages and increase health care costs, a combination that has led to proposals for governmental intervention. A recent study focused on the economic impact of obesity on the statewide economy of New Mexico. It was determined that total labor income impacts are nearly $200 million, $1,660 of output income per household, and $245 of labor income per household. Obesity cost New Mexico over 7,300 jobs and cut state and local tax revenues by over $48 million. For New Mexico, impacts total over

$1.3 billion. It is expected that the impacts in different markets, such as rural and border areas, might differ substantially from that of more populated and affluent regions. Given the differences in patient and population demographics that exist between areas even within the same state, it is imperative to conduct focused studies based on specific regions. Appropriate public health policy and health care provision decisions will depend on accurate assessment of the economic consequences of obesity in those regions.

Furthermore, when analyzing trends in patient base, revenues, market size, etc., a thorough industry level analysis may include time series econometric models to determine underlying trends and interactions among many relevant factors. Econometric models provide insight as to the responsiveness of one variable to a change in another (e.g., how market demand responds to a change in per-capita personal income). These models may also allow the practice to simulate their performance under a number of different economic scenarios. It is likely that this type of analysis would be outsourced to a consulting economist who deals with larger-scale econometric models on a routine basis. However, the benefit-to-value ratio might be quite high, for example, especially if the practice avoids locating in less profitable area.

F. The Service Package and Service Process

A detailed description of your service(s) needs to be established. The service package is a grouping of physical, sensual, and psychological benefits that are purchased together as a part of the service. The type of service process that will be utilized should be determined. In particular, the choice of service design will impact the efficiency and thus costs and profits. There are three general categories of service design. The first focuses on substituting technology for people. This design process is akin to how McDonald's uses technology (fryers, ovens, conveyor belts, etc.) to make fairly standard products available to the masses. The second design process focuses on getting the customer involved. This process is seen in self-checkouts at retailers such as Home Depot and also in salad bars, etc. The third service design process involves high customer attention. This process attempts to make the experience unique to the customer and is highly customized, such as shopping at Nordstrom. Each of these designs, or a combination of them, may be utilized in the bariatric practice. Routine follow-up care (e.g., monitoring weight, blood tests, etc.) may be standardized. Having the patient conduct tests at home and send the results to the lab/facility would be an example of getting the customer involved. Physician–patient meetings to discuss particular treatment options, etc., would likely be highly customized.

In choosing an optimal mix of services, the practice must determine the range of services to be provided. Typically, the steps involved include:

- Idea development for the service package
- Service screening (including a break-even analysis)
- Preliminary design and testing (surveys, limited market tests, etc.)
- Final design (description of resources necessary to provide your service(s))

G. Economic Benefits to All

Studies have suggested that the economic benefits of bariatric surgery outweigh the costs; thus, more practices might be socially optimal. However, the costs of bariatric surgery are a concern to some. Effective cost reduction strategies are vital if payers are to be convinced of the benefits of surgery.

Hospital or health center margins are calculated as the difference between price (i.e., revenue received for service) and cost. Economists often advocate the practice of markup pricing in order to obtain optimal earnings levels. Cost thus plays an important role in any type of markup (or *cost-plus*) strategy, and identifying differences in cost determinants for related procedures is the first step in increasing margins and profitability.

The practice should be designed so as to facilitate effective cost reduction strategies. These strategies require cost analyses of each individual procedure as results for one procedure cannot necessarily be generalized to another procedure even if overall costs do not differ. Contributions of subtypes of charges do not necessarily bear a simple relationship to the overall cost of a procedure and, in fact, each procedure requires its own cost analysis. Knowledge of these charge–cost relationships has important implications for improving hospital margins. When a single price for a procedure is charged (e.g., when hospital and surgeon fees are lumped together), the organization must focus on reducing those cost components that will add most significantly to margin.

H. Quantitative Issues: Forecasting Demand and Determining Capacity

Identifying patient demographics and demand for bariatric surgery and related services is necessary before investing time and resources into starting a practice. This aspect of the business model is aimed at identifying the market forces from the demand side of health care and determining who are likely to be potential patients or "customers" of bariatric surgery and treatment. In conjunction with data on surgery (or service) costs, estimates of the economic demand for bariatric surgery may be obtained for individuals in a particular regional market. An example of a demand study is provided by Frezza and Ewing (2006). The basic steps involved in forecasting demand for bariatric services are:

- Decide what to forecast (e.g., patient visits, etc.).
- Select appropriate data.
- Select the forecasting model (e.g., moving average or ARMA).
- Generate forecasts.

Another quantitative aspect of the business model involves determining the necessary *capacity* of the facility. This component should be measured in terms of number of patients that can be served based on demand forecasts and determine appropriate input and output measures for productivity measurement.

I. Location and Supply Chain Issues

The choice of where to locate the practice should be identified based on a number of relevant factors. While much of the location choice is subjective in nature, business models have identified several dominant location factors that should be considered in the service location decision. These factors are:

- Proximity to sources of supply (or ease in which supplies may be delivered)
- Proximity to customers
- Proximity to sources of employees
- Community considerations
- Site considerations
- Quality of life issues

Experts in operations management often utilize a factor rating model to compare alternative sites. The usefulness of these models relies on accurately weighting the location factors. The facility location decision should complement the practice's supply chain strategy in order to take advantage of cost savings and information sharing between the practice and its suppliers, outsource partners, and other strategic alliances.

J. Office Business

With the change in the way in which we practice and the corresponding increase in insurance-related issues, surgeons need to be aware of overhead analysis when opening a bariatric practice. There are multiple publications and books to assist surgeons in learning about business models from a surgical point of view. However, in order to implement successful business models in their practices, surgeons must increase their business knowledge.

Today, a surgeon is considered the manager of his or her practice and therefore must learn to act like a manager, just as if he or she were the manager of typical company. The first thing to start in a bariatric practice is a method to improve office collections. Co-payments can be quite high, and some patients pay over $300 for a surgical weight management evaluation. Patients need to know that they have to pay the co-payment just like they have to pay a dental co-payment, for example. Unfortunately, patients are not accustomed to paying for physician time and labor; therefore, they often ignore this aspect in their care and treatment plan. If the co-payment or payment for the visit is not collected prior to the visit, most of the time the payment gets lost and the surgeon loses revenue.

Additionally, whenever the surgeon sees a patient for the first time for a high grade visit, such as in the bariatric clinic, he or she can charge for a consultation for a new patient, which is CPT code 99245. The surgeon can also charge for an additional hour for an additional 30 minutes accordingly (CPT code 99355 for 1/2 hour or 99354 for 1 hour).

Recently, more surgeons are charging a fee when the surgery is scheduled. For instance, charging a nominal fee such as $250 to $500 would decrease the payment after surgery. Scheduling payments in this manner would help alleviate potential cold feet before the surgery so that the surgeon does not lose an opening in his or her daily activity. Front-loading payment, whenever feasible, is always a good business practice.

In today's office environment, every practice needs to be aware of embezzlement. Little has been reported or done to avoid embezzlement. Physicians do not usually implement proper internal controls. It is very important that jobs and duties in the office are divided among various employees. No one person needs to be in charge of collections, deposits, and recalculated with the number of visits and number of co-payments. It is very important to give vacation to employees as this time can be used to check if income increases in their absence. More can be found in recent publications. It is very important that the surgeon knows his or her bariatric practice. One of the most important things to know is what type of surgery is going to be performed, why the surgery is better than the alternatives, and the practices position in the community. All of the requirements for insurance need to be known and filed accordingly with a very well-written letter sent to the insurance company.

Given that so many people are having bariatric surgery today, surgeons need to know their leverage and create leverage within the community or within their practice. Of course, after creating leverage, surgeons need to know how to fast track approval. The first thing is to know what type of requirements the insurance company has and analyze the approval. Table 11.1 shows the importance of knowing the steps to fast track insurance approval. Table 11.2 reports our preoperative evaluation needed before surgery but this will not matter unless the office has a multidisciplinary team with a dietitian, a physiatrist, and other professionals. The 6-month diet is important. Certain insurance companies require a 1- or 5-year follow-up on patients before approving them for surgery. Medical evaluation is important to make sure that nothing is overlooked or missed. Flexibility is important to know when to change the procedure but it is very important to be consistent in procedures, as well.

Cost-effectiveness and analyzing the environment for the patient is important to point out how well this operation can be performed. It can also be cited how much the effect of bariatric surgery has impacted the state economy.

Table 11.1. Fast track insurance: Important points.

A multidisciplinary team
6-month diet
Comprehensive medical evaluation
Flexibility and consistency
Analyze each patient's indications and their cost-effectiveness
Long-term monitoring and benefits
Appeal letter

Source: Frezza EE. Six steps to Fast Track Insurance Approval for Bariatric Surgery. Obesity Surgery 2006; 16:651–663.

Table 11.2. Example of preoperative order to clear the patient medically before scheduling surgery.

Pre-op Surgery Order for Bariatric Surgery

Patient Name:_____

The above named patient will be undergoing Laparoscopic Roux-en-Y Gastric Bypass or Laparoscopic Adjustable Gastric Banding surgery. The tests below are required prior to the patient undergoing surgery. Please fax the following test results to my office ASAP. Thank you for your prompt attention to this matter.
Psychologist evaluation (psychiatrist)
EGD (adjustable band only)
Manometry (adjustable band only)

Sleep apnea test/sleep study test

H-Pylori (lab)
Complete metabolic panel/AIC level
CBC w/diff
Chest x-ray
EKG
Echocardiogram
Pulmonary function tests
Gallbladder ultrasound (if applicable)
Ultrasound of the leg to rule out deep venous thrombosis
Cardiologist clearance (performed by a *Specialist* only)
Pulmonary clearance (performed by a *Specialist* only)
Nutritionist evaluation (performed on initial office visit)

Source: Frezza EE. Six steps to Fast Track Insurance Approval for Bariatric Surgery. Obesity Surgery 2006; 16:659–663.

A good appeal letter with appropriate references also needs to be reported to help the office in case there is a denial (Table 11.3). In the office, some patients want to pay out-of-pocket but he or she does not have the money; therefore, it is important to have the appropriate paperwork to drive the patient toward either home equity or a loan. This has been discussed in the literature and it is beneficial to have the material on hand.

K. Conclusion

Running a medical practice is a business and running a bariatric practice is even more difficult. Physicians should be the managers of their practice and understand what it takes to make their practice financially sound and clinically successful.

Table 11.3. Example of a letter to send to insurance company for appeal.

Patient Name: _____
MRN: _____
DOB: _____

Date:
Insurance Company:
Fax:
Attn: Utilization Review Department
RE: Patient
Insured:
ID#:
Group#:

Procedure Code:
Type of Procedure
Procedure Fee:

Diagnosis:
ICD9 Codes:

Dear Medical Director:

This is an appeal letter on patient _____. We submitted the first letter a few months ago (see attachment). In this letter, we looked at the patient and we evaluated the patient thoroughly. He/She is a _____ -year-old female/male with a _____ body frame and weight of _____ pounds. Her/His basic metabolic index is _____. She/He has been overweight since she was a child; therefore, both her/his quality of life and life expectancy will be decreased if nothing is done.

She/He has been on several supervised and non-supervised diets and despite this, her/his quality of life has both been good and has worsened; therefore, she/he is a good candidate for a surgical management consult. We also notice that with her/his BMI, she/he is going to have problems with her/his life expectancy; therefore, something needs to be done to control her/his weight. As you know, her/his death rate is going to be much higher than other peoples. Obesity causes 300,000 deaths per year in America. She/He has a strong history of morbid obesity and comorbid disease in her/his family. Her/His comorbidities include _____.

I believe that the patient, due to the fact that she/he has been obese since childhood, is a good candidate for weight management control. The surgery for morbid obesity will benefit this patient by increasing her/his quality and length of life. Lately, several articles have been published on this subject, including:

Buchwald H. Bariatric surgery for morbid obesity: health implications for patients, health professionals, and third party payers. J Amer Coll Surg 2005;593–604.
Buchwald H. Surgical options. J Fam Pract 2005;(Suppl).

Chistou NV, Sampalis JS, Liberman M, et al. Surgery decreases long-term mortality, morbidity and health care use in morbidly obese patients. Ann Surg. 2004;240:416–423.

Maggard MA, Shugarman LR, Suttorp M, et al. Meta-analysis: surgical treatment of obesity. Ann Int Med 2005;142(7): 547–559.

Pories WJ, Swanson MS, MacDonald KG, et al. Who would have thought it? An operation proves to be the most effective therapy for adult-onset diabetes mellitus. Ann Surg 1995;222:339–350.

Torgerson JS, Sjostrom L. The Swedish Obese Subjects (SOS) Study: rationale and results. Int J Obes Relat Metab Dicord 2001;25(Suppl 1):S2–S4.

I would be more than glad to provide you with a copy of these articles. These articles describe that the impact of weight loss surgery has increased life expectancy and quality of life in more than 65% of patients.

I hope that you reconsider the patient, Mr./Mrs. _____, for the appropriate weight loss surgery. Please feel free to contact me if you have any further questions.

Thank you again for allowing me to take care of this patient.

Source: Frezza EE. Six steps to Fast Track Insurance Approval for Bariatric Surgery. Obesity Surgery 2006; 16:659–663.

L. Selected References

Baum C, Ford W. The wage effects of obesity: a longitudinal study. Health Econ 2004;13:885–899.

Frezza EE. Six steps to fast track insurance approval for bariatric surgery. Obesity Surg 2006;16(5):659–663.

Frezza EE. A plan to establish a private-pay bariatric surgery in the U.S.A. Obesity Surg 2006;16(1):110–111.

Frezza EE. Overhead analysis in a surgical bariatric practice. JLAST 2006;16(4):390–393.

Frezza EE. Avoiding embezzlement in the bariatric practice office. Obesity Surg 2006;16(10):1397–1398.

Frezza EE. Knowing your bariatric practice. What's your insurance fee? What's your leverage? Obesity Surg 2006;16(7):942–944.

Frezza EE. The business of surgery. Norwalk, CT: Cine-Med Publishing, 2007.

Frezza EE. How to improve front desk and office collection in a bariatric practice. Brief communication. Obesity Surg 2005;15(9):1352–1354.

Frezza EE, Ewing BT. Who seeks bariatric surgery? A comparison of patient demographics. Society of American Gastrointestinal Endoscopic Surgeons, Poster Session, Dallas, TX, April 2006.

Frezza EE, Wachtel MS. Practicing medicine in a new environment: what can we learn from the business managers? J Med Pract Mgmt 2006;22(1):52–54.

Frezza EE, Wachtel M, Ewing BT. The economic impact of morbid obesity on the state economy: an initial evaluation. Surg Obesity Rel Dis 2006;2:504–508.

Frezza EE, Wachtel MS, Ewing BT. Bariatric surgery costs and implications for hospital margins: comparing laparoscopic gastric bypass and laparoscopic gastric banding. Surg Laparoscop Endoscop Percut Tech. *In press*.

Must A, Spadano J, Coakley EH, et al. The disease burden associated with overweight and obesity. JAMA 1999;282:1523–1529.

Reid RD, Sanders NR. Operations management: an integrated approach. New York: John Wiley & Sons, 2005.

Statistical Abstract of the United States, 2007. Washington, DC: U.S. Census Bureau.

Wolf AM. What is the economic case for treating obesity? Obes Res 1998;6(Suppl 1): 2S–7S.

Acknowledgment: Bradley T. Ewing acknowledges financial support from the Center for Healthcare Innovation, Education and Research.

II. Techniques

12. Roux-en-Y Gastric Bypass

Robin P. Blackstone

> Medicine is a most difficult art to acquire.
> —Sir William Osler

A. Indications

The Roux-en-Y gastric bypass (RYGBP) is based on the principles of restrictive and malabsorptive bariatric operations. First performed by Mason and Ito in 1966, it has evolved into the centerpiece bariatric operation for the resolution of comorbid disease and excess weight in the United States. Two critical changes to the operation have contributed to its current reputation: Griffen modified the loop gastrojejunostomy to a Roux-en-Y in 1977 and Wittgrove and colleagues reported the laparoscopic approach in 1994. Essential steps for successful completion of this operation involve:

1. Creating a small pouch out of the larger stomach
2. Attaching a length of jejunum for egress of food out of the restrictive pouch
3. Creating an opening through which digestive effluent may combine with food for digestion to occur

B. Approach: Open versus Laparoscopic

Public perception is that laparoscopic surgery is less invasive, but there are additional advantages for a surgeon evolving from an open to a laparoscopic approach. Pfuzziferi in a randomized, prospective trial with 3-year outcomes showed an advantage for laparoscopic surgery related to length of hospital stay, incisional pain, return to work, and a markedly decreased rate of incisional hernia between open cases (39%) vs. laparoscopic (5%, $p < 0.01$). An additional comparison by Nguyen between open ($n = 6,065$) and laparoscopic ($n = 16,357$) Roux-en-Y gastric bypass procedures performed in a university setting demonstrated that major complications such as an anastomotic leak, venous thrombosis, and pneumonia were increased in patients with an open approach. Seventy-three percent of the cases in this setting were laparoscopic, which reflects the growth of this type of access. Both studies show no difference between the open and laparoscopic approach in regard to resolution of comorbid disease, quality of life, or excess weight loss.

C. Patient Position and Room Setup

The patient is prepared in the preoperative area with intravenous fluid rehydration, intravenous antibiotics, and subcutaneous anticoagulation. The operating room table should be able to sustain the weight of the patient being operated, capable of being manipulated into reverse Trendelenburg, and covered with gel foam padding to reduce the incidence of cutaneous pressure neuropathies. Antithrombolic stockings are started prior to the institution of anesthesia. Patients can be positioned with legs in a supine or lithotomy position (Fig. 12.1).

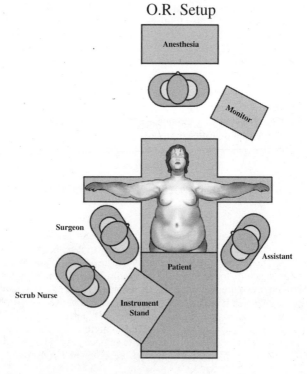

Figure 12.1. Operating room set-up.

D. Operative Procedure

This procedure is one of the most complex performed laparoscopically, and is associated with a significant learning curve. Initial cases should be proctored and focused on patients with lower BMI and less complex comorbid disease. Efficient operating room times usually run between 90 and 120 minutes.

1. Establish the pneumoperitoneum

Most commonly a Veress needle is placed through the abdominal wall just below the left rib cage. Insufflation to 15 mmHg will usually be adequate to achieve visualization. Once the shape of the abdomen has been established with an initial insufflation of 4 L, trochars can be placed under direct vision.

2. Placement of trochars

A local anesthetic is used to infiltrate the skin of the abdomen prior to incision. The first trochar (12 or 5 mm) should be placed with a zero degree camera under direct visualization one handbreadth below the xiphoid/manubrial junction and slightly to the left of midline to avoid the ligamentum teres. Using the xiphoid as the starting point will usually result in the midline trochar being too low, especially in male patients with deep diaphragms. In patients with a previous midline or right upper quadrant incision, the first trochar should be placed in the left upper quadrant in the mid-clavicular line after first establishing where the point of the V will be in the midline. For the remainder of the operation an angled (30- or 45-degree) scope is used. Subsequent trochars are placed in the mid-clavicular and anterior axillary line on both sides in the shape of a V. The steepness of the V will be determined by the body shape and configuration once insufflation is complete. An additional 5-mm trochar is placed just to the left of the xiphoid where the liver retractor can be placed. The use of blunt trochars should be used to decrease the incidence of incisional hernia. Examination of the abdomen should be carried out (Fig. 12.2).

3. Retraction of the liver

The liver is often very large and is an impediment to visualization of the esophageal hiatus. Use of a Nathanson-type retractor through an epigastric port (usually 5 mm) may be necessary for extremely large or heavy livers; otherwise a toothed grasper attached to the diaphragm usually will be sufficient. Over time the liver "fatigues" and tends to fold over the retractor. The liver should be retracted so that both the Angle of His and the pars flaccida can be seen in the field.

4. Creation of gastric pouch

Opening the peritoneum over the diaphragmatic muscle at the Angle of His allows the surgeon to visualize the angle of dissection of the pouch. A thin band of connective tissue in front of the first short gastric protects the superior and

Port Placements

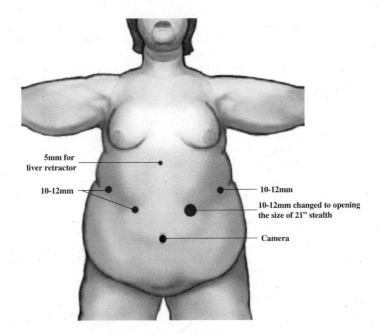

5mm for
liver retractor

10-12mm

10-12mm

10-12mm changed to opening
the size of 21" stealth

Camera

Figure 12.2. Laparoscopic port placement.

medial edge of the spleen during the dissection. Dissection of the gastrohepatic ligament directly on the stomach wall, decreases blood loss, and preserves the function of the vagus nerve. Using an ultrasonic dissector may be preferred. A small 2- to 3-cm opening along the lesser curve below the anterior fat pad and above the first vessel is the correct place to access the lesser sac. If a balloon has been placed into the stomach to size the pouch, the linear stapler should be closed just below the bottom of the balloon but the linear stapler should not be fired until the balloon is removed. Sequential division of the stomach using the anterior fat pad as the anterior guide to the creation of the pouch and angling the stapler up to the angle of His should result in a 15- to 20-cc pouch. It is critical to change direction of the stapler from left (first firing) to right (subsequent firings), angling directly to the angle of His to avoid injury to the spleen and avoid including the fundus of the stomach in the pouch (Figs. 12.3–12.5).

5. Gastrojejunostomy

Three established methods of creating the gastrojejunostomy have been described, and many variations exist. Trade-offs exist between the rate of stricture and

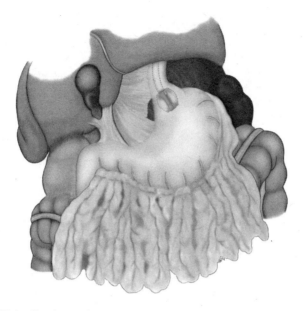

Figure 12.3. Gastric pouch construction.

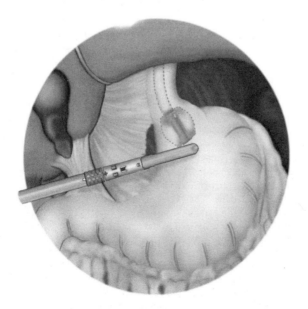

Figure 12.4. Gastric pouch construction.

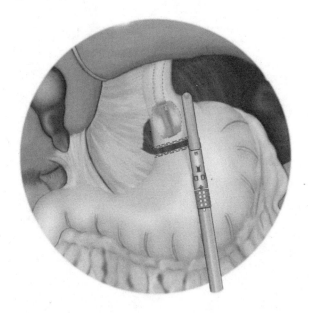

Figure 12.5. Gastric pouch construction.

long-term dilation of the anastomosis with weight regain. These issues are among the considerations in deciding which technique to offer patients.

    a.   Circular stapler technique. Two common variations involve the way in which the anvil is placed in the gastric pouch (Figs. 12.6–12.12).

Intra-abdominal: The circular stapler can be introduced into the stomach by making an enterotomy and drawing the anvil through the wall of the stomach pouch prior to completing division of the stomach. This has the advantage of being able to use a larger-diameter stapling device (25 mm with a 15-mm internal opening diameter), but leaves an anterior gastric enterotomy to be closed, which is at risk for leakage if postoperative gastric distention occurs.

Pulldown: An angiocatheter is placed through the wall of the abdomen under direct visualization and a pull wire introduced into the abdomen. An endoscope is introduced into the pouch through which a snare has been placed flush against the end of the endoscope. The scope is positioned against the stomach wall posterior to the staple line and held firmly. The snare is pushed against the wall of the pouch and can be visualized in the abdomen, where a short burst of cautery will create a small opening through which the snare is extruded. The snare captures the end of the pull wire and the wire is brought up out of the mouth and attached through the center of the anvil and looped over the mushroom cap of the anvil. The anvil is guided into the posterior pharynx by the anesthesiologist and then a jaw lift is performed and the anvil drawn gently down into the pouch and through the small opening of the pouch. Once the roux limb has been brought into the upper abdomen, the circular stapler is introduced into the abdomen,

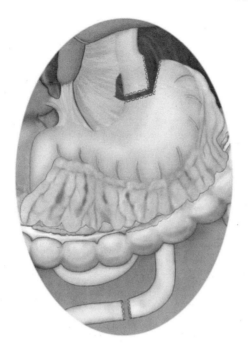

Figure 12.6. Circular stapler technique.

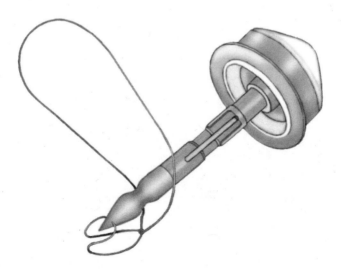

Figure 12.7. Circular stapler technique.

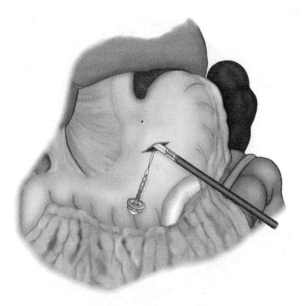

Figure 12.8.   Circular stapler technique.

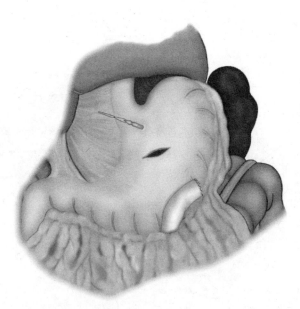

Figure 12.9.   Circular stapler technique.

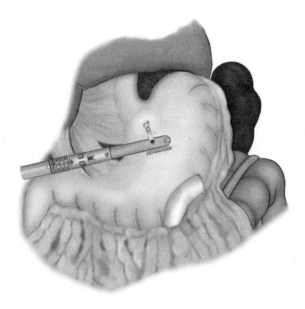

Figure 12.10.   Circular stapler technique.

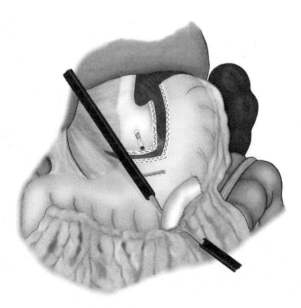

Figure 12.11.   Circular stapler technique.

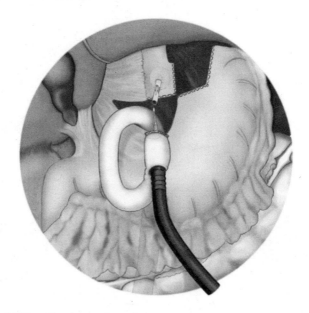

Figure 12.12.   Circular stapler technique.

usually through the left mid-clavicular port site after dilation of the port site from 12 to 25 mm using Hegar dilators. The circular stapler is placed into the lumen of the jejunum and the needle of the stapler is extruded through the wall of the jejunum, approximately 4 cm from the cut end. The needle is docked to the anvil under direct vision checking to assure the tissue below the stapler is not included and rotating the roux limb to lie in a "candy cane" configuration. The stapler is fired and removed by pulling backward and turning the stapler in a half circle. The end of the roux limb is closed with a linear stapler. The integrity of the "donuts" of resected tissue can be inspected, but the ultimate judge of adequate closure is the leak test performed at the end of the procedure. The bent end of the candy cane should not be very long, and undesired excess jejunum can be excised while closing the end of the roux limb. At the conclusion of the procedure the left mid-clavicular port site is irrigated with antibiotic irrigation and the fascial stitches are tied.

Technical Note: Occasionally the anvil will seem to be difficult to pull down, letting go of the pull wire and allowing the anvil to "bounce" up the esophagus and then gently pulling again slowly will usually solve this problem. Most of the time the anvil is caught at the cricopharyngeal junction and sometimes taking down the balloon of the tracheostomy tube will be necessary to facilitate passage of the stapler. The liver retractor can also be a barrier to passage of the anvil (see Fig. 12.4).

   b.   Hand-sewn technique. The hand-sewn anastomosis requires advanced laparoscopic suturing technique. It is the least expensive option and has the added benefit of decreasing the infection rate in the port site through which the circular stapler is placed. The anastomosis is usually created anterior on the gastric pouch. A posterior, running layer is created between the staple line of the gastric pouch and antimesenteric side of the roux limb using 3-0 polyglactin suture. Enterotomies are made in the gastric pouch and jejunum and a second posterior running, full thickness layer is made and continued anteriorly. Prior to completion of the anastomosis a 34 F bougie is passed carefully through the anastomosis and the anterior inner (full thickness) and outer (seromuscular) layers are completed.

c. Linear stapler technique. After the roux limb is brought into the upper abdomen a small enterotomy is made in both the roux limb and pouch. The linear cutter is placed and fired for a length of about 1.5 cm. The enterotomy is closed from either end using an absorbable Vicryl suture (3-0 polyglactin) until the last stitch is ready to be tied down. The 30 F endoscope is passed through the anastomosis and the stitch is tied down using the endoscope as a "stent." A second layer of absorbable suture is required to complete the anastomosis.

d. Checking for anastomotic leak. Prior to completing the operation all anastomosis, regardless of technique, are checked by obstructing the roux limb with an endo-glassman clamp. The endoscope is positioned under direct vision just above the gastrojejunal anastomosis. Air is insufflated through the endoscope into the gastrojejunal anastomosis with air until tense insufflation of the roux limb above the clamp occurs. Flooding the intra-abdominal field with water will reveal any air leak, which signals a leak of the anastomosis. Additional stitches can be taken until the test yields a satisfactory result. Early in a surgeon's experience opening to correct the leak may be the best option. False tests can result if tense insufflation is not achieved.

6. Jejunojejunostomy

The jejunojejunostomy is constructed using a toothed grasper or a stitch to stabilize both the stapled end of the antimesenteric surface of the biliopancreatic limb and the roux limb at the desired length. Small enterotomies are made with an ultrasonic dissector (cautery may result in a larger defect) and an anastomosis of 45–70 mm is created between the two limbs. Firing in two opposite directions may decrease the incidence of obstruction. The enterotomy is closed with an additional horizontal firing of the linear stapler or by hand sewing the defect closed. All staple lines should be visually inspected to assure closure and evaluate the opening size. Careful attention should be paid to the way the roux limb lies, and if "kinking" is observed a Bolin stitch can be taken to allow the roux limb to lie more naturally (Fig. 12.13).

7. Roux limb: antecolic vs. retrocolic

a. Retrocolic. The lesser sac is opened through the pars lucida and a 1-cm white Penrose drain placed behind the stomach. The colon is reflected cephalad and the ligament of Treitz is identified. A 2- to 4-cm opening is made above the pancreas in the mesocolon and the Penrose drain is

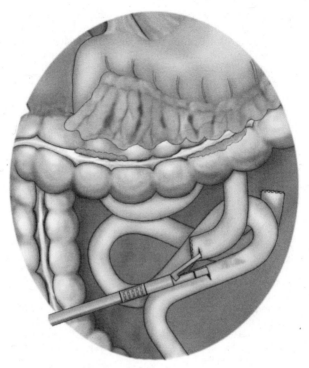

Figure 12.13.   Jejunojejunostomy.

retrieved. The jejunum is divided approximately 15 cm from the ligament
of Treitz using a linear stapler and the mesentery is "notched" on the side
of the roux limb. A 100-cm (Routine) or 150-cm (long limb) is measured,
and then the jejunojejunostomy is created. Once the jejunojejunostomy
has been completed, the end of the roux limb is attached to the Penrose
drain and placed carefully (pulling only on the Penrose drain) through
the mesocolon and behind the stomach. Replacing the colon in its usual
position in the abdomen the Penrose drain is gently retracted back from
the lesser sac drawing the roux limb gently into the upper abdomen where
it should lie without slipping back under the stomach. The roux limb is
brought up through the lesser sac and out through the gastrohepatic ligament, allowing the gastrojejunal anastomosis to be created where the back
wall of the anastomosis lies on the soft tissue of the ligament, creating a
"patch" of soft tissue that heals quickly.

b.   Antecolic. Division of the omentum down to the anterior colon wall
using an ultrasonic dissector is made. The colon is then reflected into
the upper abdomen and the ligament of Treitz identified. A 30- to 35-cm
biliopancreatic limb is created to facilitate bringing the 65- to 70-cm roux
limb anterior to the colon. The roux limb is brought into the upper abdomen through the notched defect in the omentum. The total length of the
bypassed jejunum is approximately equal to the retrocolic approach.

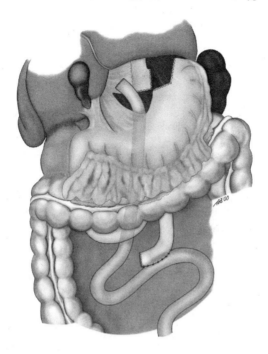

Figure 12.14.   Retrocolic Roux-en-Y gastric bypass.

Debate continues over the best approach to use, particularly as it affects the incidence of internal hernia. Carmody and DeMaria reported on 785 patients who had an internal hernia after gastric bypass. The lowest rate of internal hernia occurred in 3/542 patients with a retrocolic approach and closure of all defects with permanent suture (0.55%). In 6/107 patients who had a retrocolic approach without closure of defects (5.6%, $p < 0.0001$). In the same study 12/136 patients with the antecolic approach had internal hernia (8.81%, $p < 0.0001$) (Fig. 12.14).

8. Closure of defects

Closure of all mesenteric defects using *permanent* suture should be done prior to completing the operation in an attempt to decrease the incidence of internal hernia.

E.   Selected References

Buchwald H, Avidor Y, Braunwald E, et al. Bariatric surgery: a systematic review and meta-analysis. JAMA 2004;292(14):1724–1737.

Carmody B, DeMaria EJ, Jamal M, et al. Internal hernia after laparoscopic Roux-en-Y gastric bypass. Surg Obes Relat Dis 2005;1(6):543–548.

Gagner M, Garcia-Ruiz A, Arca MJ, et al. Laparoscopic isolated gastric bypass for morbid obesity. Surg Endosc 1999;13:S6.

Griffen WO, Young VL, Stevenson CC. A prospective comparison of gastric and jeju-noileal bypass procedures for morbid obesity. Ann Surg 1977;186:500–507.

Higa KD, Boone KB, Ho T, et al. Laparoscopic Roux-en-Y gastric bypass for morbid obesity: technique and preliminary results of our first 400 patients. Arch Surg 2000;9:1029–1033.

Mason EE, Ito C. Gastric bypass in obesity. Surg Clin North Am 1967;47:1345–1352.

Murr MM, Gallagher SF. Technical considerations for transabdominal loading of the circular stapler in laparoscopic Roux-en-Y gastric bypass. Am J Surg 2003;185(6): 585–588.

Nguyen NT, Hinojosa M, Fayad C, et al. Use and outcomes of laparoscopic versus open gastric bypass at academic medical centers. J Am Coll Surg 2007;205(2):248–255.

Puzziferri N, Austrheim-Smith IT, Wolfe BM, et al. Three-year follow-up of a prospec-tive randomized trial comparing laparoscopic versus open gastric bypass. Ann Surg 2006;243(2):181–188.

Schauer PR, Ikramuddin S, Gourash W, et al. Outcomes after laparoscopic roux-en-Y gastric bypass for morbid obesity. Ann Surg 2000;232(4):515–529.

Schauer PR, Ikramuddin SI, Hamad G, et al. The learning curve for laparoscopic Roux-en-Y gastric bypass is 100 cases. Surg Endosc 2003;17:212–215.

Wittgrove AC, Clark GW, Tremblay LF. Laparoscopic gastric bypass, Roux-en-Y: prelimi-nary report of five cases. Obes Surg 1994;4:353–357.

Acknowledgments:

All figures in this chapter are reprinted with permission, ©1999–2007 Ethicon Endo-Surgery, Inc. All rights reserved.

Disclosure:

Dr. Blackstone holds an appointment as associate clinical professor of surgery at the University of Arizona College of Medicine-Phoenix. She is a consultant for Ethicon Endosurgery and Allergan Medical. Scottsdale Bariatric Center par-ticipates in FDA clinical trials for Enteromedics and Allergan Medical and in protocols with the National Institutes of Health. She is a member of the board of directors for the Surgical Review Corporation and has served on the Bariatric Surgical Review Committee of the Surgical Review Corporation for 4 years. She was elected to the Executive Committee of the American Society for Metabolic and Bariatric Surgery in 2007. She is a founding member of the Board of Direc-tors of the Obesity Action Coalition.

13. Lap-Band® and Adjustment Schedule

Dean J. Mikami

A. Indication and Description

In June 2001, the Lap-Band® System (Allergan, Inc., Irvine, CA) became the first FDA-approved laparoscopic adjustable gastric band (LAGB) for patients 18 years and older in the United States. Indications for LAGB placement are the same for any bariatric procedure (BMI >35 with one or more obesity-related comorbidity or BMI >40). LAGB is a restrictive procedure in which an inflatable silicone band is placed around the upper part of the stomach. The band is placed just below the gastroesophageal junction and secured with sutures. The adjustment port is then tunneled through the abdominal wall and secured to the anterior abdominal wall fascia. The creation of a smaller stomach pouch results in restriction of the amount of food that can be consumed at one time. LAGB increases the time it takes for the stomach to empty. Weight loss is achieved by limiting food intake, reducing appetite, and slowing digestion. There are currently three Lap-Band sizes (Fig. 13.1) available in the United States: 9.75/10, VG, and the AP.

B. Patient Position and Room Setup

1. Position the patient supine with both arms out.

    The patient should be secured to the OR table to prevent the patient from sliding downward during reverse Trendelenburg positioning. We use a split leg OR table with the operating surgeon standing between the patient's legs.
2. The video monitors are placed at the patient's left and right shoulder.
3. Sequential compression devices should be placed on before anesthetic induction.
4. An appropriate antibiotic should be given prior to incision.

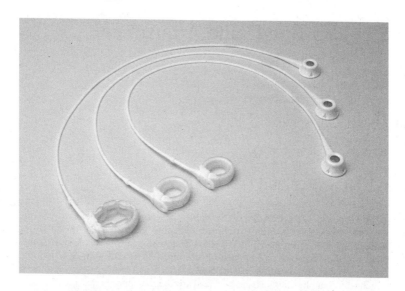

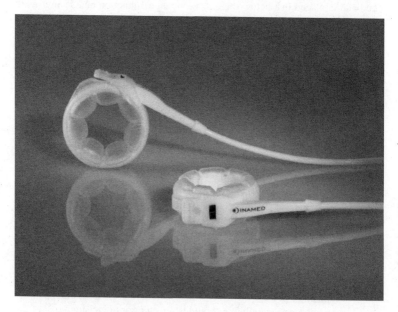

Figure 13.1. **a** Lap-Band VG, 10.0 and 9.75. *Source*: Reprinted with kind permission from Allergan, Inc. **b** Lap-Band AP. *Source*: Reprinted with kind permission from Allergan, Inc.

C. Trocar Position and Choice of Laparoscope

1. The surgeon stands between the patient's legs and the assistant surgeon stands on the patient's left side.
2. A Veress needle is then inserted at the left mid-clavicular position, below the left costal margin. The first trocar (15-mm) is inserted at this site (Fig. 13.2, scarlet dot).
3. A 30-degree, 5- or 10-mm laparoscope is then place above the umbilicus (Fig. 13.2, gray dot).
4. Two additional 5-mm trocars are placed (Fig. 13.2, white dots).
5. A Nathanson liver retractor is placed at the epigastrium (Fig. 13.2, green dot).

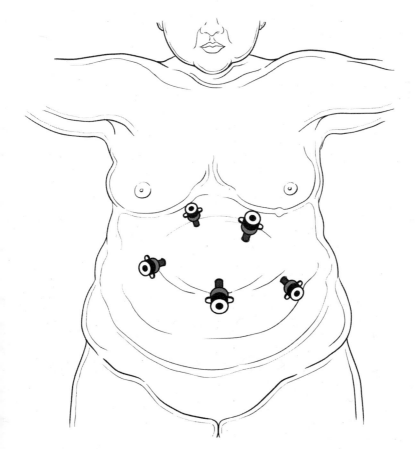

Figure 13.2. Trocar position for laparoscopic adjustable band placement.

D. Operative Technique

1. Pars flaccida technique (preferred).
2. Dissection of the angle of His, freeing the gastrophrenic peritoneal attachments to expose the left crus.
3. Creation of a 15–20 cc pouch.
4. Posterior dissection just below the crura.
5. Anterior fixation of the fundus and anterior gastric wall over the band (Fig. 13.3).
6. Complete deflation of the band at time of placement.
7. The end of the band is brought through a port site.
8. The access port is placed and sutured to the anterior rectus sheet with permanent suture.

E. Advantages

1. Low mortality rate
2. No division of stomach or small bowel
3. Adjustable
4. Reversible
5. Low postoperative complication rate
6. Low malnutrition rate
7. Shorter hospital stay

F. Disadvantages

1. Slower weight loss
2. Less weight loss as compared with combined restrictive/malabsorptive operations (gastric bypass, duodenal switch)
3. Requires an implantable medical device
4. Band slippage, erosion, and esophageal dilatation
5. Access port malfunctions
6. Requires ongoing patient monitoring and adjustments for optimal weight loss

G. Complications

1. Mortality rate: 0.05%
2. Total complication rate: 11%
3. Major complications

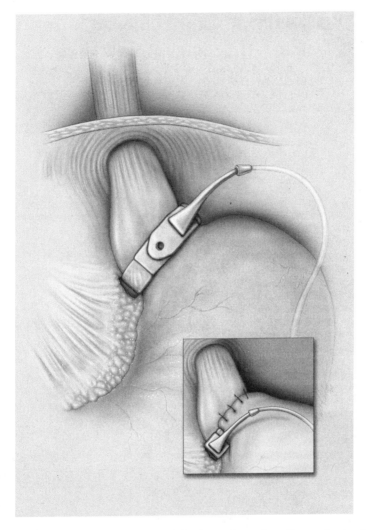

Figure 13.3. Anterior fixation of the fundus and gastric wall over the band. *Source*: Reprinted with kind permission from Allergan, Inc.

    a.   Band slippage (3.1–8.1%)
    b.   Band erosion (0.2–2%)
    c.   Esophageal dilatation (6.6–10%)

4.   Access port problems (0.11–3.0%)

H. Results: US Data

1. 12-month Excess body weight loss percentage (EBWL%): 33–50
2. 24-month EBWL%: 45–63
3. 36-month EBWL%: 44–65
4. 48-month EBWL%: 58–62
5. 60-month EBWL%: 50–65

I. Lap-Band Adjustments

1. Typically starts 6 weeks after surgery
2. Weight loss goal is 0.5 to 1 kg per week
3. Can be done in the office or with fluoroscopy depending on the depth of the access port
4. The adjustment goal is to achieve a sensation of prolonged satiety
5. Adjustment can be done every 4 to 6 weeks or as needed
6. 9.75- and 10-cm band (max volume: 4 cc)

   a. 0.5–1 cc added at first adjustment
   b. 0.3–0.5 cc added or removed at subsequent adjustments

7. VG and AP Standard (APS) (max volume: 10 cc), AP Large (APL) (max volume: 14 cc)

   a. 3–4 cc added at first adjustment
   b. 1–1.5 cc added or removed at subsequent adjustments

8. Consider adding saline

   a. Inadequate weight loss
   b. Rapid loss of satiety after meals
   c. Hunger between meals

9. Adjustment not required

   a. Adequate rate of weight loss (>0.5 kg and <1 kg per week)
   b. Eating a reasonable range of food
   c. No negative symptoms

10. Consider removing saline

    a. Persistent nausea and emesis
    b. Wheezing, coughing spells, and choking
    c. Difficulty with a broad range of foods

J. Selected References

Allen JW. Laparscopic gastric band complications. Med Clin North Am 2007;91.

DeMaria EJ, Jamal MK. Laparoscopic adjustable gastric banding: evolving clinical experience. Surg Clin North Am 2005;85:773–787.

Favretti F, O'Brien PE, Dixon JB. Patient management after LAP-BAND placement. Am J Surg 2002;184:38s–41s.

Halloway JA, Forney FA, Gould DE. The Lap-Band is an effective tool for weight loss even in the United States. Am J Surg 2004;188:659–662.

Ponce J, Paynter S, Fromm R. Laparoscopic adjustable gastric banding: 1014 consecutive cases. J Am Coll Surg 2005;05:529–535.

Provost DA. Laparoscopic adjustable gastric banding: an attractive option. Surg Clin North Am 2005;85:789–805.

14. Laparoscopic Duodenal Switch

Manish Parikh, Michel Gagner,
and Alfons Pomp

A. Introduction

Laparoscopic biliopancreatic diversion with duodenal switch (BPD-DS) is one of the most effective weight loss procedures currently available. Both short- and long-term weight loss exceed that of any other bariatric operation. BPD-DS involves a 150- to 200-cc sleeve or vertical gastrectomy, a duodenoileal anastomosis, and a long Roux-en-Y with a 150-cm alimentary limb and a 100-cm common channel (Fig. 14.1). The key features of this operation are that the lesser curvature, antrum, pylorus, first portion of the duodenum, and vagal innervation are all spared, while parietal cell mass is reduced, thus allowing a better digestive behavior while decreasing the likelihood of the dumping syndrome and marginal ulceration. Furthermore, by placing the ileoileal anastomosis 100 cm proximal to the ileocecal junction (instead of 50 cm, as in the classic Scopinaro BPD), metabolic disturbances and the number of surgical revisions for malnutrition or diarrhea are considerably less.

B. Indications/Special Preoperative Preparation

1. All patients should meet NIH criteria for obesity surgery (namely, BMI >40 kg/m^2 or >35 kg/m^2 with obesity-related comorbidities). Particularly the superobese (BMI >50 kg/m^2) and super-superobese (BMI >60 kg/m^2) are excellent candidates for this procedure, as BPD-DS provides superior weight loss outcomes in these patients compared with gastric bypass. Other indications and contraindications are listed in Table 14.1.
2. EGD to exclude gastric or duodenal pathology, including *Helicobacter pylori* infection.
3. If *H. pylori* is present, patients are treated prior to surgery.
4. Upper GI series if the patient has had a prior bariatric procedure.
5. Medical clearance.
6. Psychiatric evaluation and instruction by registered dietitian/nutritionist.
7. Screening colonoscopy if the patient is above age 50.
8. Evaluation for obstructive sleep apnea (if applicable).
9. Clear liquid diet the day prior to surgery.

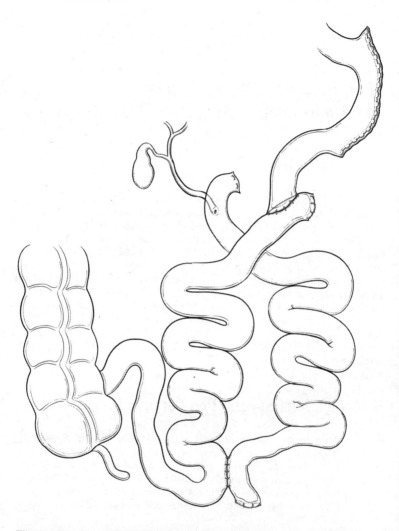

Figure 14.1. Lap BPD/DS: Sleeve gastrectomy, duodenoileostomy and a long Roux-en-Y with a 150 cm alimentary limb and 100 cm Common channel.

C. Patient Position and Room Setup (Fig. 14.2)

1. Alpha-Max table (Maquet; Rastatt, Germany) with foot-plate attachments
2. French, split-leg position with the legs abducted, but not flexed, and properly secured

Table 14.1. Indications and contraindications for Lap BPD-DS.

Indications
- BMI >40 kg/m^2 or >35 kg/m^2 with obesity-related comorbidities
- Superobese (BMI >50 kg/m^2) and super-superobese (BMI >60 kg/m^2)
- Patients who want to avoid the dietary/volume restrictions of the gastric bypass
- Patients considering gastric bypass but who require high-dose anti-inflammatory medications (e.g., for severe arthritis)
- Patients who require periodic surveillance of their stomach
- Patients who have failed vertical-banded gastroplasty, gastric banding, or gastric bypass

Contraindications
- Patients who are bedridden
- Patients who are vegetarian (patients need to ingest at least 80–100 g protein daily)
- Patients with prior colon resection (may be prone to developing diarrhea)
- Patients with severe gastroesophageal reflux (may be better served with gastric bypass)
- Patients with inflammatory bowel disease
- Patients with prior gastrectomy

3. The surgeon stands between the patient's legs, the first assistant (liver retractor and camera holder) stands on the patient's right, and the second assistant stands on the patient's left.

D. Trocar Placement

1. Seven trocars total (Fig. 14.3)

   a. 10-mm trocar at umbilicus (we prefer the open technique to enter the peritoneal cavity)—diagnostic laparoscopy is then performed with the 10-mm 30-degree laparoscope
   b. Two 10-mm trocars—left epigastric paramedian position (optics) and right subcostal position in the mid-clavicular line (liver retraction)
   c. Two 5- to 15-mm Versaports (Tyco Healthcare, Norwalk, CT)—right mid-clavicular line just superior to umbilicus and left mid-clavicular line, four fingerbreadths inferior to the costal margin
   d. 5- to 12-mm Versaport in the subxiphoid position
   e. 5-mm port in left anterior axillary line lateral to the Versaport

2. A second insufflator is attached to optimize pneumoperitoneum (15 mmHg carbon dioxide)

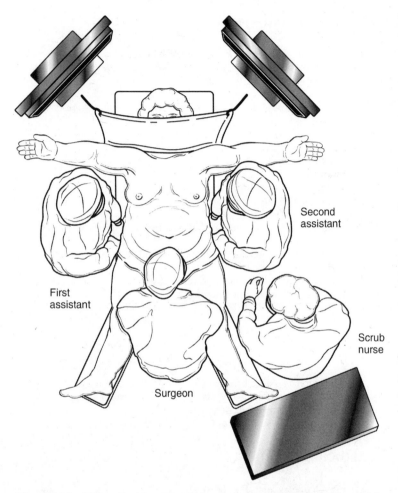

Figure 14.2. Patient Position: The patient is in the split-leg position with the surgeon between the patient's legs, the first assistant (camera operator/liver retractor) on the patient's right and the second assistant on the patient's left.

E. Technique

We prefer to start with the sleeve gastrectomy rather than the distal ileoileostomy because occasionally patients cannot tolerate pneumoperitoneum and may require a shortened procedure. In these cases, performing a sleeve gastrectomy alone permits an effective, abbreviated procedure without compromising the patient. Several months later (after significant weight loss has taken place), the patient may return for "second-stage" completion duodenal switch.

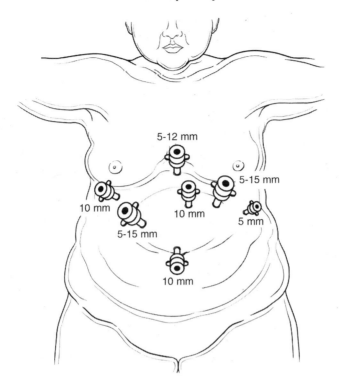

Figure 14.3. Trocar Positions.

1. Sleeve gastrectomy

a. The patient is placed in steep reverse Trendelenburg position and the table is tilted right side down to optimize visualization of the gastroesophageal junction.

b. The laparoscope is placed through the 10-mm left epigastric paramedian trocar. If the stomach is distended the anesthesiologist should place an orogastric tube to decompress the stomach; this tube must be removed as soon as the stomach is decompressed to avoid any problems during subsequent stapling.

c. A 10-mm liver retractor (fan-type retractor) is placed through the right subcostal port to retract the liver anteriorly and expose the entire stomach and gastroesophageal junction. The surgeon's working ports are the subxiphoid Versaport and the left subcostal Versaport. The second assistant retracts the omentum laterally with a bowel grasper through the 5-mm left lateral trocar.

d. Dissection begins along the distal greater curvature by dividing the branches of the gastroepiploic artery near the gastric wall with the ultrasonic scalpel. The greater curvature is devascularized in this manner proximally to the level of the left crus (including division of the short gastric vessels). The second assistant's grasper is frequently repositioned superiorly to maximize retraction. Exposure while dividing the short gastric vessels and dissecting near the left crus is often difficult. Helpful maneuvers include:

- Place the second assistant's grasper on the lateral fold of the omentum (in the mid-gastrosplenic ligament) and retract this laterally toward the spleen.
- Temporarily increase the pneumoperitoneum to 20 mmHg.
- Place the patient in maximal reverse Trendelenburg position.
- Tilt the patient more toward the right side.
- Ask the anesthetist to give an additional dose of paralytics.
- Position the second assistant on the posterior fundus and retract this toward the patient's right side.
- Occasionally an additional 5-mm trocar is required to retract the perigastric fat and adequately expose the gastroesophageal junction.

e. All posterior attachments to the pancreas must be freed, taking care not to injure the splenic artery. Placing the second assistant's graspers on the posterior fundus and retracting this toward the patient's right shoulder exposes these attachments. It is important to divide these attachments prior to stapling because these attachments can tear and create significant bleeding. However, one must not be too aggressive near the lesser curvature because the blood supply to the sleeve will come from the lesser curvature vasculature only.

f. Now the left crus can be visualized by lifting the stomach anteriorly. The left crus and gastroesophageal junction must be completely exposed. The ligament attaching the stomach and diaphragm must be divided. The anterior perigastric fat just to the left of the gastroesophageal junction must be cleared to minimize tissue thickness during subsequent stapling. However, avoid dissecting to the right of the gastroesophageal junction because of risk of injury to the vagus nerve. If the patient has a significant hiatal hernia, this should be reduced because failure to recognize/repair herniated fundus may lead to weight loss failure and reflux after sleeve gastrectomy.

g. Next the remainder of the greater curvature is liberated distally to 2 cm beyond the pylorus. The second assistant retracts the greater curvature anteriorly toward the patient's right shoulder. The surgeon's left hand grasps the fat of the gastrocolic ligament (via the right mid-clavicular Versaport) and retracts it caudad. The surgeon's right hand manipulates the ultrasonic scalpel. The remainder of the gastrocolic ligament between the antrum and gastroepiploic arcade is divided with the ultrasonic scalpel.

h. Instrument palpation is used to confirm the anatomic position of the pylorus. Approximately 6 to 8 cm proximal to the pylorus (at the level of the "crow's foot," just distal to the incisura) the sleeve gastrectomy is begun along the greater curvature (Fig. 14.4). Initiating the sleeve less than 6 cm proximal to the pylorus may compromise the antrum and could lead to gastric emptying problems.

i.   The surgeon's left hand holds the 4.8-mm linear stapler (60 mm in length) through the right mid-clavicular Versaport. The second assistant retracts the body of the stomach toward the patient's left side. The stapler should be positioned such that at least 2 cm of anterior stomach serosa is visible between the stapler and lesser curvature.

j.   The first two firings of the stapler are performed, aiming approximately 2 cm away from the lesser curvature. These firings should be done slowly because the stomach is thickest in this area. Additional sutures may be required if the tissue is too thick for the stapler. We routinely use buttress material (Bioabsorbable Seamguard; Gore, Flagstaff, AZ) similar to the Maxon suture (United States Surgical, Norwalk, CT), which is sandwiched between, over, and below the anterior and posterior gastric wall. This bioabsorbable material reduces staple-line hemorrhage and possibly the leakage rate.

k.   The anesthesiologist inserts a 60 Fr orogastric bougie and, under laparoscopic vision, the bougie is aligned medially along the lesser curvature into the duodenum. Two bowel graspers can be used to help direct the bougie posteriorly into the sleeve toward the pylorus. Inserting the

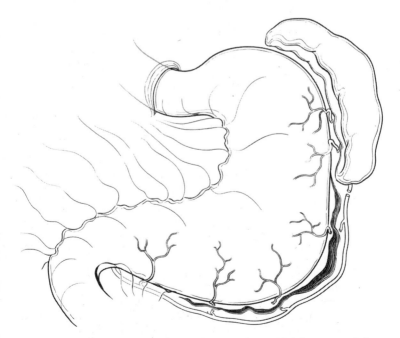

Figure 14.4. Mobilization of the branches of the gastroepiploic artery and short gastric vessels in preparation for the sleeve gastrectomy.

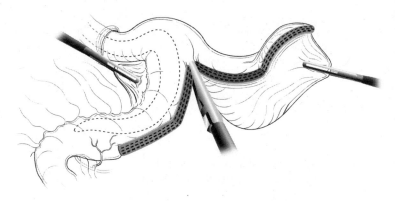

Figure 14.5. Posterior and antero-lateral retraction around the bougie.

bougie after the first two stapler firings helps align the bougie along the lesser curvature (Fig. 14.5). For all duodenal switch cases, we currently use the 60 Fr bougie to ensure enough volume of the stomach to permit adequate protein intake. (For primary sleeve gastrectomy we use a smaller bougie, 32–40 Fr.)

l. The remainder of the sleeve gastrectomy is completed by sequential firings of the 4.8-mm linear stapler along the bougie toward the angle of His (Fig. 14.6). Although we have used the 3.5-mm linear stapler in the past, we believe that it is safest to use the 4.8-mm linear stapler for the entire sleeve gastrectomy due to the thick stomach in these morbidly obese patients. The differences in hemostasis between the two staplers are no longer seen with the routine use of the buttressing Seamguard material. The surgeon's right hand holds the stapler via the left mid-clavicular Versaport and aims toward the left crus; the surgeon's left hand (via the subxiphoid Versaport) grasps the anterior wall of the stomach (or the perigastric fat) and retracts this toward the patient's right side. The second assistant holds the posterior wall of the stomach and retracts this toward the patient's left side. A total of five to six staple firings are typically required to complete the sleeve. The anesthesiologist must pay careful attention that the bougie does not retract during stapling to prevent the tip of the bougie from being incorporated into the staple line.

m. Next, the anesthesiologist removes the bougie. We prefer to place figure-of-eight 3-0 Maxon (monofilament absorbable) sutures at the apex of the sleeve gastrectomy (the area most prone to developing leak), at the intersections of the staple lines (also prone to suboptimal healing) and at the most distal end of the staple line (thickest part of stomach). The second assistant can retract the stomach toward the patient's right side to help expose the apex of the sleeve.

n. If there is any doubt about the integrity of the staple line, a methylene blue test should be performed prior to proceeding to the next stage. The

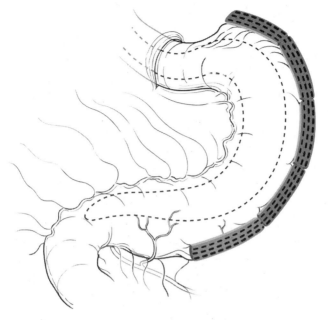

Figure 14.6. The laparoscopic sleeve gastrectomy is created by sequential firings of the 4.8-mm stapler along a 60-Fr bougie towards the angle of HIS.

anesthesiologist inserts an 18 Fr orogastric tube. The surgeon clamps near the pylorus and the anesthesiologist injects methylene blue mixed with saline through the tube. Approximately 120 cc are required to distend the sleeve. Another option is to insert a gastroscope and check for leak (and intraluminal bleeding) via air insufflation; this latter option is used less often because of the tendency of air to pass through the pylorus and distend the small bowel.

o. The right mid-clavicular trocar site is enlarged, the abdominal wall is dilated with an atraumatic clamp (the circular stapler will be introduced through this site later), a large impermeable bag is introduced and the specimen is extracted. Grasping the end of the sleeve and pulling it out progressively may make extraction easier and require less abdominal wall dilation.

2. Duodenal transection and preparation for duodenoileostomy

a. The pylorus and first portion of duodenum are palpated. Any remaining branches between the gastroepiploic arcade and the antrum/pylorus are divided with the ultrasonic scalpel, proceeding toward the inferior aspect of the first portion of the duodenum. Typically, the dissection extends to just beyond the vascular complex inferior to the pylorus. It is important to avoid hemostatic clips in this area (especially on the duodenal side) to prevent having clips interfere with the staple line. Any duodenal adhesions from prior cholecystectomy must be divided at this time.

b.   The retroduodenal and supraduodenal tissue are dissected free with the ultrasonic scalpel. The second assistant retracts the stomach laterally and anteriorly so the surgeon can see both the greater curvature and the posterior stomach for the retroduodenal dissection. The gastroduodenal artery, which lies posteriorly between the first and second portion of duodenum, marks the distal aspect of dissection.

c.   Using a 10-mm right-angle dissector, a 1-cm window (enough to accommodate a linear stapler) is made posterior and superior to the duodenum, medial to the common bile duct (Fig. 14.7). Ideally, the supraduodenal window is between the serosa of the duodenum and the pyloric branches of the right gastric artery, thus maximizing blood supply to the subsequent anastomosis.

d.   The duodenum is transected with a 3.5-mm Endo-GIA linear stapler (60 mm in length; Tyco Healthcare, Norwalk, CT) buttressed with Bioabsorbable Seamguard leaving a 2- to 5-cm duodenal cuff (typically via the left mid-clavicular Versaport; Fig. 14.8). Sometimes, the right mid-clavicular Versaport provides a better angle for transection. The second assistant retracts the antrum toward the patient's left side to facilitate this. The Seamguard buttressing material obviates the need to oversew the duodenal stump.

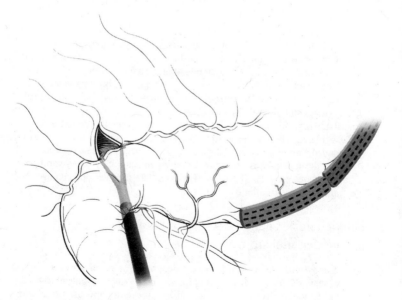

Figure 14.7. Peridoudenal dissection.

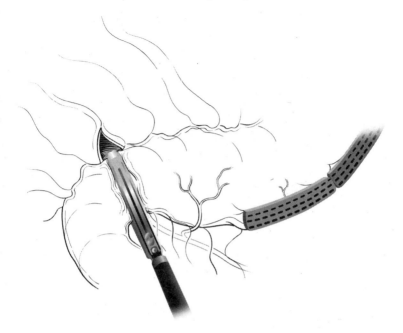

Figure 14.8. Duodenal transection with 3.5-mm linear stapler (60 mm in length).

e. If the surgeon is faced with a scenario where he or she is unable to complete the supraduodenal window, an alternate method is to transect the inferior two thirds of the duodenum with the linear stapler, complete the supraduodenal window, and then transect the remaining duodenum with another firing of the stapler.

f. We prefer to use a circular stapler for the duodenoileostomy, specifically the CEEA 21 (Tyco Healthcare, Norwalk, CT). The CEEA 25 is too large for the ileum and frequently tears the ileum during insertion. The 21 anvil is delivered transabdominally through the right mid-clavicular trocar site. The 21 anvil is problematic to deliver through the proximal duodenal stump using the modified nasogastric tube-anvil apparatus commonly used for gastric bypass because it does not flex and traverses the pylorus only with some difficulty.

g. The ultrasonic scalpel is used to remove 1 to 2 cm of the proximal duodenal staple line and the base of the 21 anvil is placed into the duodenal lumen. Once the anvil is in place, it is secured with a 3-0 Prolene pursestring suture (Fig. 14.9).

h. Next the surgeon must assess the ability of the ileum to be brought toward the duodenum antecolic and in a tension-free manner. Particularly in patients with bulky omentum, one must divide the omentum

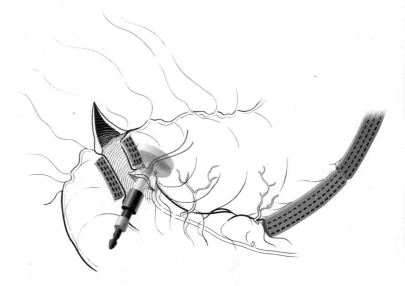

Figure 14.9. 21-mm anvil inserted into proximal duodenum and secured with 3–0 Prolene purse-string suture.

along its right lateral third to facilitate subsequent passage of the ileum toward the duodenum. It is important that the right side of the omentum (and not the left side, as commonly done in gastric bypass) is divided because an oblique line runs from the ileocecal valve toward the pylorus.

3. Small bowel measurement

a. The surgeon and first assistant move to the patient's left side. The patient is placed in the Trendelenburg position and then tilted left side down to aid in exposure of the ileocecal region.

b. With the laparoscope in the left epigastric paramedian port and the surgeon's working hands in the subxiphoid and umbilical ports, the distal small intestine is measured from the ileocecal valve using a 50-cm umbilical tape. Flat 5-mm forceps (Dorsey, Karl Storz; Tutlingen, Germany) are used to avoid serosal tears during measurements. Any adhesions that prevent proper measurement of the small intestine (e.g., prior lower abdominal or pelvic surgery) must be divided. The umbilical tape should be kept on the antimesenteric side during measurements. We prefer umbilical tape for these measurements because it is a more reliable method of measuring small intestine vs. estimating distances with a bowel grasper.

c. At 100 cm proximal to the ileocecal valve, clips are placed on the ileal mesentery (to mark the site of anastomosis of the future common channel). Another 150 cm is measured proximally from this point (future alimentary limb). Here, a window is made in the ileal mesentery with a 10-mm right-angle clamp. It is best to not dissect directly on the bowel wall, as the mesentery advances over the intestinal wall in the morbidly obese. Instead, make the window in the mesentery approximately 1 cm away from the bowel wall.

d. The ileum is transected with a 2.5-mm linear stapler (45 mm in length is adequate) buttressed with Bioabsorbable Seamguard (via the left mid-clavicular Versaport). The ultrasonic scalpel is used to divide another 1 to 2 cm of mesentery between the two ends of bowel. Dividing more than 1 to 2 cm of mesentery is unnecessary and places the subsequent anastomosis at risk of becoming ischemic.

e. The grasper remains on the distal bowel (with the umbilical tape) to maintain proper orientation. The staple line and buttress material are completely excised from the distal ileum to permit entry of the 21-mm circular stapler. The umbilical tape is then removed. Care is taken to make sure there is no twisting of the mesentery or misidentification of bowel limbs by running the bowel again from the ileocecal valve proximally to the transected (and opened) ileum.

4. Duodenoileal anastomosis

a. A suture is attached to the spike of the CEEA 21 for easy retrieval. The CEEA 21 is secured to a plastic camera drape (for wound protection) with a Steri-Strip and is introduced via the right mid-clavicular trocar site.

b. Three graspers are used to triangulate the opened end of ileum: two are placed at the 2:00 and 10:00 positions and a third grasper is placed at the 6:00 position adjacent to the mesentery.

c. The stapler is gently maneuvered into the distal ileal enterotomy and advanced cephalad in a clockwise manner toward the duodenal cuff containing the anvil. The first two graspers are removed. The grasper at 6:00 remains in place to prevent the stapler from coming out of the bowel. It is critical that the ileum is brought toward the duodenum (and not vice versa) under minimal or no tension. The omentum needs to be divided to facilitate this, as described earlier.

d. The first assistant moves between the patient's legs and the surgeon remains on the patient's left (second assistant remains on the patient's right to retracting the liver anteriorly).

e. The white plastic perforator is advanced through the antimesenteric wall of ileum approximately 6 to 7 cm distal to the opened ileum. The spike is removed by grasping the suture attached to the spike. The anvil (in the duodenum) is then united with the stapler (Fig. 14.10). It is important that there is no tissue between the ileum and duodenum and that there is no pinching of the bowel wall (which can create an obstruction later).

f. The stapler is fired and an end-to-side anastomosis is created. The CEEA 21 is not a flipped-top; therefore, two to three rotations of the stapler are required in conjunction with counter-traction on the antrum in order to pull the CEEA through the anastomosis.

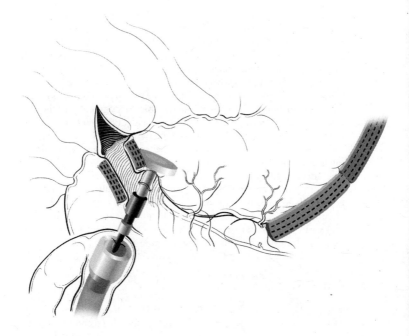

Figure 14.10.   The anvil of the CEEA 21 and the stapler are united.

g. Next, the Steri-Strip holding the wound protector is removed and the CEEA is removed from the trocar site while advancing the wound protector over the tip of the stapler in order to prevent the stapler from contacting the wound.

h. The surgeon returns between the legs and the first assistant returns to the patient's right side. The right mid-clavicular Versaport is re-inserted.

i. The open ileal limb is inspected for bleeding—any oozing emanating from the enterotomy may indicate bleeding from the duodenoileostomy and must be further evaluated. If there is no bleeding from the open limb, a 2.5-mm linear stapler (45 mm in length) buttressed with Bioabsorbable Seamguard (via the subxiphoid or left mid-clavicular trocar) is used to transect the blind limb. The tips of the stapler must be in the ileal mesentery to ensure that the opened ileum has been completely closed (otherwise a leak can occur into the mesentery). The specimen is extracted from the right mid-clavicular trocar site.

j. The duodenoileostomy staple line (including the upper and lower corners) is reinforced with a running 3-0 Maxon suture. We prefer monofilament absorbable sutures for this because permanent sutures (e.g., Silk sutures) have been associated with marginal ulcers and strictures. One helpful maneuver to provide adequate exposure of the superior corner (where leaks are most prone to occur) is to place the second assistant's graspers on the antrum and retract this toward the patient's left lower quadrant in order to pull the anastomosis toward the midline. To facilitate exposure of the posterior aspect of the staple line, the second assistant should grasp the posterior antrum and gently retract this toward the patient's right shoulder.

k. Next, the anesthesiologist inserts an 18 Fr orogastric tube just proximal to the anastomosis and then instills approximately 120 cc methylene blue mixed with saline with a Tumi syringe. Simultaneously, the surgeon clamps the ileum distal to the duodenoileostomy. The area around the anastomosis is irrigated with saline to help identify any methylene blue. Once the test has been completed and no leak has been identified, the gastric sleeve is completely aspirated and the orogastric tube is removed.

5. Distal ileoileostomy

a. The surgeon and first assistant return to the patient's left side and the laparoscope is placed through the left epigastric paramedian trocar. The table is tilted left side down and the patient is placed in slight Trendelenburg position.
phoid and umbilical port to run the alimentary limb from the duodenoileostomy distally to the level of the previously placed clips on the ileal mesentery (at 100 cm proximal to the ileocecal valve).

c. We prefer the "M" triple-staple technique, which is a completely stapled anastomosis that provides a large patent anastomosis while avoiding the risk of narrowing the bowel lumen during closure of the enterotomy (Fig. 14.11). The clips on the ileal mesentery are removed.

d. An enterotomy is made with the ultrasonic scalpel on the antimesenteric side of the marked ileum. Another enterotomy is made approximately 1 to 2 cm away from the stapled end of the proximal ileum. The stapled proximal ileum (biliopancreatic limb) should be on the patient's left and the alimentary limb should be on the patient's right side. Again, one must take care that there has been no twisting of the mesentery and that both staples are fired on the antimesenteric border to avoid ischemia.

e. The 2.5-mm linear stapler (60 mm in length) is introduced through the subxiphoid Versaport, aiming toward the pelvis. It is best to insert the larger jaw of the stapler into the proximal ileum (larger diameter) and the smaller jaw into the distal ileum (narrower). A standard side-to-side anastomosis is created between the biliopancreatic limb and the last 100 cm of distal ileum.

f. Through the same enterotomy, the linear stapler (2.5, 60 mm in length) is then fired between the alimentary limb and the common channel. A third firing of the 2.5-mm linear stapler (via the left mid-clavicular Versaport) closes the enterotomy transversely. The specimen is removed without contaminating the wound. An alternate option for enterotomy closure is to close the enterotomy with a running 2-0 silk suture, either in one or two layers.

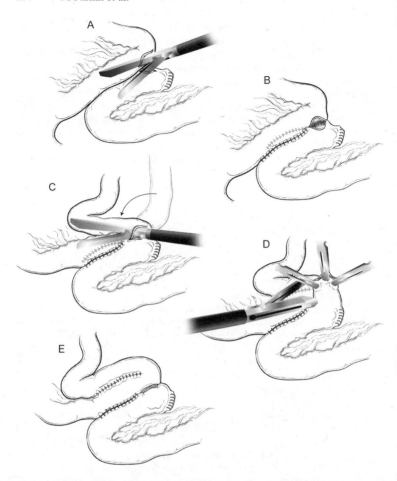

Figure 14.11. Creating the ileoileostomy using the "M" stapling technique. A standard side-to-side anastomosis is created between the biliopancreatic limb and the last 100 cm of distal ileum to create the common channel (A–B). Through the same enterotomy, the linear stapler (2.5, 60 mm in length) is first between the alimentary limb and the common channel (C). A third firing of the 2.5-mm linear stapler closes the enterotomy transversely (D–E).

6. Closure of mesenteric defects

a. We recommend complete closure of all mesenteric defects to avoid internal hernias and their associated complications. With the same position (surgeon and first assistant on the patient's left side), the ileoileostomy mesenteric defect is closed with a running 2-0 silk suture

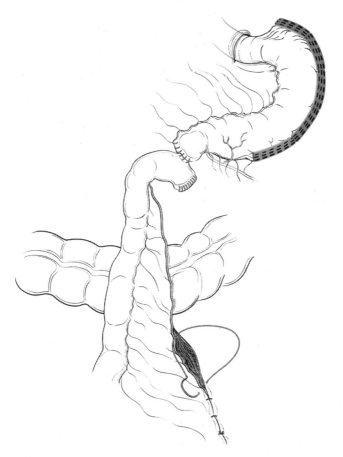

Figure 14.12. Closure of Petersen's defect.

(24 cm in length). We prefer to incorporate the serosa of the ileum in the last stitch of this closure.

b. The surgeon then returns between the legs in order to close Petersen's defect (Fig. 14.12). The patient is placed in slight reverse Trendelenburg position. Sometimes, it is necessary to insert an additional 5-mm trocar in the left lower quadrant to optimize suturing angles.

c. The omentum is retracted superiorly to the transverse colon. The first assistant grasps the epiploic appendage of the transverse colon and retracts this cephalad. Now this space between the transverse colon mesentery and the ileal mesentery should be completely exposed, and this defect is closed with a running 2-0 silk suture.

   d. We prefer to close this from the patient's left side because there is a wider space on the left and closure from the left side permits visualization of the ligament of Treitz and helps the surgeon avoid catching proximal jejunum in the closure. The final stitch should approximate the transverse colon serosa to the ileum serosa, because mesenteric fat closure alone may eventually (with significant weight loss) enlarge and lead to an internal hernia. It is imperative to completely close these defects, especially at the root of the mesentery, because a small defect may be more susceptible to incarceration than the initially large patent defect.

7. Closure

   a. The sleeve gastrectomy staple line, duodenoileostomy, and ileoileostomy are all inspected for any evidence of bleeding or leakage. The biliopancreatic limb must be coming from the patient's left side and the alimentary limb and the common channel must be on the patient's right side.

   b. We do not routinely place any drains or a nasogastric tube.

   c. All fascial defects larger than 5 mm are closed with a suture-passing device (Karl Storz, Tutlingen, Germany) with 0-Vicryl sutures. The umbilical site is usually closed under direct vision with a #1 Prolene suture. Skin incisions are closed with subcuticular absorbable monofilament sutures.

F. Alternate Techniques

   1. Although we prefer to use the circular stapler (CEEA 21) for construction of the duodenoileostomy, there are several alternatives.

      a. Linear stapler (side-to-side anastomosis, 3.5-mm blue cartridge). Place one jaw of the linear stapler in the ileum, bring it up to the duodenum, and place the second jaw into the duodenotomy and then fire the stapler. The enterotomy may be closed with a running suture. The downside of this approach is that a large enterotomy inevitably results, which needs to be closed primarily.

      b. Hand-sewn technique: two layers, end-to-end or end-to-side. This has a difficult learning curve and is associated with the longest operative time.

      c. Hand-assisted: through a small midline incision. This may be useful for surgeons early in their learning curve. However, this approach may provide fewer benefits (e.g., wound complications, analgesic requirements, postoperative recover, etc.) compared with the completely laparoscopic approach.

   2. Originally, most surgeons avoided the circular stapler because of the difficulty experienced placing the anvil into position, especially

when trying to pass the anvil through the pylorus (using the modified nasogastric tube apparatus). We have adapted our technique to position the anvil via duodenotomy (followed by Prolene pursestring suture to secure the anvil in place), and this has significantly reduced our operative time.

3. Alternate techniques for the ileoileostomy include hand-sewn (associated with longer operating times) and the double-stapled technique (biliopancreatic limb to common channel and closure of enterotomy). Our concern with the latter technique is that this may narrow the common channel during closure of the enterotomy, particularly due to the smaller-diameter ileum.

4. The most critical factor that results in a leak at the duodenoileostomy is exaggerated tension at the anastomosis. Maneuvers to eliminate tension at the anastomosis include:

    a. Division of the omentum needs along its right lateral aspect.
    b. Mobilization of the right colon.
    c. Division of blood vessels superior to the pylorus: one must be cautious because this may compromise the blood supply to the anastomosis.
    d. We have not found retrocolic duodenoileostomy to be necessary; the preceding maneuvers should ensure a tension-free anastomosis. Moreover, we generally avoid retrocolic construction due its association with increased incidence of internal hernias.

5. The surgeon should always consider the two-stage approach in the high-risk superobese or in the patient who cannot tolerate prolonged pneumoperitoneum, has extensive intra-abdominal adhesions, or lacks adequate working space despite higher pneumoperitoneum pressures. A two-stage approach (laparoscopic sleeve gastrectomy followed by completion duodenal switch 6–12 months later) has the advantages of technical facility, shorter operative times, and interval weight loss between stages, which in turn results in decreased morbidity in this high-risk group.

6. It is advisable to keep the total operative time to less than 4 hours to avoid the attendant risks (pulmonary, thromboembolic, and rhabdomyolysis) of prolonged general anesthesia, especially in the high-risk bariatric patient.

G. Postoperative Care

1. Patients are closely monitored for at least 6 hours.
2. Patients are placed on continuous positive airway pressure (CPAP) if sleep apnea is present or suspected.
3. Maintenance intravenous fluids are continued to ensure urine output of at least 0.5 to 1 cc/kg/hour.
4. Early ambulation is critical. The majority of our patients ambulate the very evening of surgery.
5. We use postoperative upper gastrointestinal contrast studies selectively:

     a.   In cases of any intraoperative technical difficulties (e.g., positive methylene blue test requiring additional sutures)

     b.   For patients who manifest signs and symptoms concerning for leak (e.g., fever greater than 38.5 °C, tachycardia, tachypnea, somnolence and failure to thrive, etc.)

6.   Patients usually require an intravenous patient-controlled analgesic pump for the first 2 days.

7.   They receive clear liquids on the first postoperative day. If they do well, their Foley catheters are removed and they are weaned off the intravenous fluids.

8.   Patients are advanced to a pureed diet the next day.

9.   Our nutritionist sees all patients postoperatively, and their dietary recommendations are reviewed.

10.   Patients are usually discharged home by the third postoperative day on a pureed diet and oral analgesics.

11.   Patients are seen 4 weeks after discharge. They receive follow-up nutritional counseling for a protein-enriched diet, and are given twice-daily multivitamins, oral calcium supplements, iron, and fat-soluble vitamins.

12.   Patients with intact gall bladders are prescribed ursodiol 300 mg twice daily for 6 months for gallstone prophylaxis.

13.   At 3 months postoperatively, a thorough nutritional evaluation is performed, including serum levels of iron, ferritin, vitamin B_{12}, folate, albumin, PTH, calcium, phosphorus, alkaline phosphatase, zinc, selenium, lipids, vitamins A and D, total protein, and hematology panels.

H. Selected References

Baltasar A, Bou R, Miro J, et al. Laparoscopic biliopancreatic diversion with duodenal switch: technique and initial experience. Obes Surg 2002;12:245–248.

Buchwald H, Avidor Y, Braunwald E, et al. Bariatric surgery. A systematic review and meta-analysis. JAMA 2004;292:1724–1737.

Comeau E, Gagner M, Inabnet W, et al. Symptomatic internal hernias after laparoscopic bariatric surgery. Surg Endosc 2005;19:34–39.

Consten E, Gagner M, Pomp A, et al. Decreased bleeding after laparoscopic sleeve gastrectomy with or without duodenal switch for morbid obesity using a stapled buttressed absorbable polymer membrane. Obes Surg 2004;14:1360–1366.

Feng J, Gagner M, Pomp A, et al. Effect of standard vs. extended Roux limb length on weight loss outcomes after laparoscopic Roux-en-Y gastric bypass. Surg Endosc 2003;17:1055–1060.

Gagner M, Inabnet W, Pomp A. Laparoscopic sleeve gastrectomy with second stage biliopancreatic diversion and duodenal switch in the superobese. In: Inabnet W, DeMaria E, Ikramuddin S. Laparoscopic bariatric surgery. Philadelphia: Lippincott Williams & Wilkins, 2005:143–150.

Gagner M, Matteotti R. Laparoscopic biliopancreatic diversion with duodenal switch. Surg Clin North Am 2005;85:141–149.

Gastrointestinal Surgery for Severe Obesity. NIH Consensus Statement, March 25–27, 1991;9:1–20.

Marceau P, Hould F, Simard S, et al. Biliopancreatic diversion with duodenal switch. World J Surg 1998;22:947–954.

Prachand V, Davee R, Alverdy J. Duodenal switch provides superior weight loss in the super-obese (BMI >50 kg/m^2) compared with gastric bypass. Ann Surg 2006;255:611–619.

Rabkin R. The duodenal switch as an increasing and highly effective operation for morbid obesity. Obes Surg 2004;14:861–865.

Rabkin R, Rabkin J, Metcalf B, et al. Laparoscopic technique for performing duodenal switch with gastric reduction. Obes Surg 2003;13;263–268.

Regan J, Inabnet W, Gagner M, et al. Early experience with two-stage laparoscopic Roux-en-Y gastric bypass as an alternative in the super-super obese patient. Obes Surg 2003;13:861–864.

15. Laparoscopic Sleeve Gastrectomy: A Staged Procedure for Super-Super Obese Patients

Kuldeep Singh

A. Indications and Rationale

Although laparoscopic bariatric surgery has evolved into a very safe and effective procedure, the super-super obese patients (BMI >60) continue to pose significant technical challenges. This translates to higher complications and poor outcomes in this group of patients, irrespective of the nature of the surgery. There seems to be a linear correlation between the outcomes and the risk of the surgery. The riskier the operation is—laparoscopic bilio-pancreatic diversion with duodenal switch (BPD-DS), laparoscopic Roux-en-Y gastric bypass (LGBP)—the more effective weight loss appears to be.

The challenges in super-superobese patients (BMI >60) are both functional as well as technical. The functional challenges include poor cardiopulmonary reserve, exercise intolerance, restrictive as well as obstructive lung disorders (translates into inability to tolerate anesthesia) and inability to ambulate.

The technical challenges are:

- Difficult access to abdominal cavity, higher pneumoperitoneum pressures
- Large and stiff abdominal wall, decreasing the maneuverability of the instruments
- Large fatty left lobe of the liver making difficult the exposure of the gastroesophageal junction and making prone to injury to organs such as liver, spleen, esophagus, and stomach
- Thick and foreshortened small bowel mesentery from fatty infiltration creating tension at anastomosis and vascular compromise of the intestine by either stretching or by attempts to lengthen by the mesenteric division

Sleeve gastrectomy was originally conceived by Marceau in 1993 as modification to partial gastrectomy in BPD. BPD-DS is a long and complex operation with significant morbidity and mortality. In order to reduce to operating times, simplify the operation into two stages and let patient lose some weight and thus decrease the complication rate, Gagner and colleagues suggested BPD-DS as a staged procedure where LSG is the first stage. Subsequent follow-up of these patients has suggested that sometimes LSG may be the only operation needed in some patients.

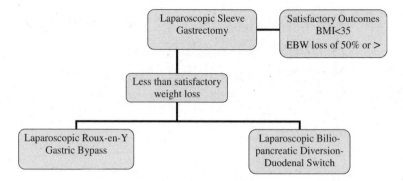

Figure 15.1. Laparoscopic sleeve gastrectomy: a staged procedure.

LSG obviates the need for infra-colic intestinal reconstruction, simplifies and shortens the procedure, and effectively reduces the comorbidities/obesity. This makes the second (malabsorptive) stage of the BPD easier and faster to accomplish, if needed. The Sleeve also makes gastric pouch reconstruction relatively easy to perform in LGBP. Its simplicity and effectiveness has led to its gaining acceptance as a staged procedure (Fig. 15.1).

B. Patient Positioning and Room Setup

1. The patient is placed supine with arms on the sides on the arm boards. The feet rest on a foot board fixed to the bed. There is a folded blanket under the knees, the legs and thighs are strapped to the bed. A Foley catheter is placed in aseptic fashion.
2. The video monitors are on either side of the patient's shoulders.
3. SQ Heparin given preop and sequential compression devices are placed on the legs.
4. Preoperative antibiotics are given.
5. Orogastric tube is placed and stomach decompressed. The tube is then replaced by size 34 Maloney Bougie. It is ensured laparoscopically that the tip of the bougie is beyond the pylorus.

C. Port Position

1. Access is obtained by using 12-mm Visiport (Covidien, Mansfield, MA) using 10-mm zero degree scope, traversing the layers of abdominal wall under vision. The ideal position for entry if left paramedian where layers are very well defined.

2. Pneumoperitoneum of 17 mm of mercury is obtained and general inspection of the abdomen is done noting the size of the liver, any injuries of entrance and other incidental findings.
3. The port position is shown in Fig. 15.2. One additional 15-mm trocar is placed in right paramedian position, one in left subcostal margin and one 5-mm trocar are inserted in the right subcostal margins. One 5-mm subxiphoid obturator is inserted and a medium Nathanson retractor (Cook Medical, Bloomington, IN) is inserted to retract the left lobe of the liver. This is held by Iron Intern retractor system (Automated Medical Product Corp, Edison, NJ) attached to left side of the side rails.
4. A 10-mm 45-degree scope is used for the surgery.

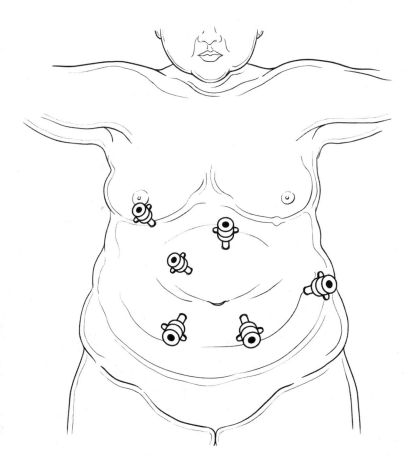

Figure 15.2. Laparoscopic sleeve gastrectomy: port placement.

D. Stage-1. Laparoscopic Sleeve Gastrectomy

1. The anatomical landmarks such as Crow's foot and gastroesophageal junction are identified. Any dimpling of the hiatus is explored by dividing the fat pad over the EG junction and hiatal hernia repaired if present.
2. Gastrocolic and gastrosplenic omentum is divided with Ligasure (Covidien, Mansfield, MA) at the greater curvature of the stomach and the stomach completely mobilized and rotated medially. Exposure of the left crus of the diaphragm ensures that the dissection is complete and pouch remains small.
3. The Crow's feet (the terminal branches of nerves of Laterjet) on lesser curvature is identified and a point diagonally opposite on greater curvature is identified as starting point for division. This is approximately 6 cm proximal to the pylorus.
4. The first stapler is fired with Endo GIA stapler of green thickness (4.8 mm) 60 mm in length, introduced through the right-sided 15-mm trocar. This thickness is needed to divide the thick pylorus and antral muscle fibers. The remaining stapler loads are fired parallel to the bougie as shown in Fig. 15.3.

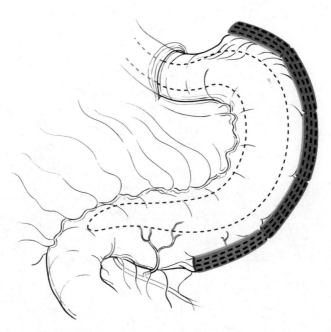

Figure 15.3. Laparoscopic sleeve gastrectomy: creation of sleeve.

5. The remainders of the firings are done with either green or blue thickness stapler load reinforced with staple-line reinforcement products.
6. Great care is taken to divide close to the bougie as adhesions to the retroperitoneum or fatty infiltration of the lesser curvature mislead to a larger sleeve.
7. The Angle of His clearly identified and stomach is divided just lateral to the left diaphragmatic crus.
8. The areas of staple line overlap or transition is oversewn with Zero Surgidac suture using Endostich instrument.
9. The pylorus is clamped and gastroscope is used to insufflate the stomach under water and areas of air leak and lamberted.
10. A size 10 flat JP is inserted and specimen removed through an enlarged 15-mm trocar site.
11. All 12- and 15-mm trocars are closed with zero Polysorb suture.

E. Stage-2. Laparoscopic Roux-en-Y Gastric Bypass or Laparoscopic Biliopancreatic Diversion—Duodenal Switch

1. Port placements are done same as one stage procedure.
2. In GBP, the stomach is transected 5 cm distal to GE junction by 60 mm long, 4.8-mm thick stapler. The Roux-en-Y reconstruction is done in usual fashion (retrocolic-retogastric linear staple technique).
3. In BPD-DS, the technique is described by M. Gagner and colleagues. Dissection and division of first portion of the duodenum is done followed by creation of duodeno-ileostomy by 25-mm EEA stapler (transoral technique). Ileoileostomy is then created by linear stapling technique creating 150 cm of alimentary limb and 100 cm of common channel. All the mesenteric defects are closed in running fashion.

F. Selected References

Gagner M, Inabnet WB, Pomp A. Laparoscopic sleeve gastrectomy with second stage biliopancreatic diversion and duodenal switch in the superobese. In: Inabnet WB, DeMaria EJ, Ikramuddin S, eds. Laparoscopic bariatric surgery, 2nd ed. Philadelphia: Lippincott Williams &Wilkins, 2005:145–150.

Gumbs A, Gagner M, Dakin G, et al. Sleeve gastrectomy for morbid obesity. Obes Surg 2007;17:962–969.

Marceau P, Biron S, Bourque RA, et al. Biliopancreatic diversion with a new type of gastrectomy. Obes Surg 1993;3:29–35.

16. Laparoscopic Staged Roux-en-Y: A Staged Procedure for Super-Super Obese Patients

Ninh T. Nguyen and Marcelo W. Hinojosa

A. Indications

Laparoscopic Roux-en-Y gastric bypass in the super-super obese (BMI >60 kg/m²) population can be challenging. Factors that contribute to the technical difficulty include male gender, android body habitus, and high BMI. Men often have an android body habitus with high content of visceral fat, which increases intra-abdominal pressure and reduces intraoperative laparoscopic visualization. In addition, android body habitus and high BMI are often associated with fatty liver disease and enlarged liver lobes that may obscure visualization of the gastroesophageal junction. All of these factors can contribute to the degree of intraoperative technical difficulty and should be weighed in the selection of appropriate patients to undergo laparoscopic gastric bypass.

Although a high BMI is not in itself a contraindication to surgery, laparoscopic gastric bypass in the super-super obese can be associated with a higher morbidity and mortality. In an effort to minimize perioperative morbidity, the concept of a two-stage operation was developed. The initial two-stage procedure consists of a sleeve gastrectomy (first stage) followed by an interval Roux-en-Y gastric bypass or duodenal switch. However, the sleeve gastrectomy can still be challenging in the super-super obese, particularly in patients with an enlarged liver from nonalcoholic steatohepatitis or liver cirrhosis obscuring visualization of the gastroesophageal junction near the angle of His. The alternative two-stage procedure is the staged Roux-en-Y, which consists of a modified Roux-en-Y operation with construction of a larger gastric pouch and a low gastrojejunal anastomosis. Construction of a large gastric pouch avoids the difficult dissection of the angle of His. The construction of a low gastrojejunal anastomosis minimizes tension on the anastomosis and hence reduces the chance for leaks. In the second stage, 6 to 12 months later, the volume of the gastric pouch is reduced by performing a sleeve gastrectomy of the gastric fundus.

B. Patient Position and Room Setup

1. Position the patient supine with both arms to the side. A foot board should be placed. The patient's legs should be secured to prevent the patient from sliding during reverse Trendelenburg position.

2. Place the video monitors at the patient's left and right shoulder.
3. Place a Foley catheter.
4. The sequential compression device should be active during anesthetic induction.
5. Antibiotics should be given.

C. Trocar Position and Choice of Laparoscope

1. The surgeon stands on the patient's right side. The assistant surgeon stands on the patient's left side.
2. Place the Veress needle at the left mid-clavicular position above the umbilicus.
3. The first trocar (11-mm) is inserted at this site.
4. Four additional abdominal trocars are placed (one 12-mm and three 5-mm trocars), as shown in Fig. 16.1.
5. A 45-degree angle laparoscope should be used.

D. Laparoscopic Staged Roux-en-Y (First Stage)

1. The operation begins with construction of the jejunojejunostomy.
2. Identify the ligament of Treitz and divide the jejunum 40-cm distally with a linear stapler (blue load). The jejunum mesentery is divided with a linear stapler (gray load).
3. The Roux limb is measured at 150-cm. The base of the Roux limb is fashioned to the jejunal biliopancreatic limb. A side-to-side jejunojejunostomy is constructed using a 60-mm linear stapler (white load). The remaining jejunal defect is closed with a running, two-layer closure. The small bowel mesenteric defect is closed with a running suture.
4. The greater omentum is divided to provide an antecolic path for the Roux limb.
5. The patient is switched to a reverse Trendelenburg position.
6. The hepatogastric ligament, close to the lesser curvature of the stomach, is divided using a linear stapler (gray load). An anterior gastrotomy is made low on the lesser curvature. The 25-mm anvil is inserted transabdominally and placed through the gastrotomy and positioned on the anterior gastric wall approximately 4 or 5 cm distal to the gastroesophageal junction. The stomach is divided starting on the lesser curvature and completed on the greater curvature (Fig. 16.2a).
7. Pass the end of the Roux limb, on an antecolic path, into proximity to the gastric pouch, taking care to avoid twisting of the mesentery.
8. The gastrojejunal anastomosis is constructed with a 25-mm circular stapler. The circular stapler is inserted transabdominally and then positioned through the end of the Roux limb. The surgeon connects the anvil with the stapler to construct the gastrojejunostomy. The end of the Roux limb is closed with a linear stapler (blue load).

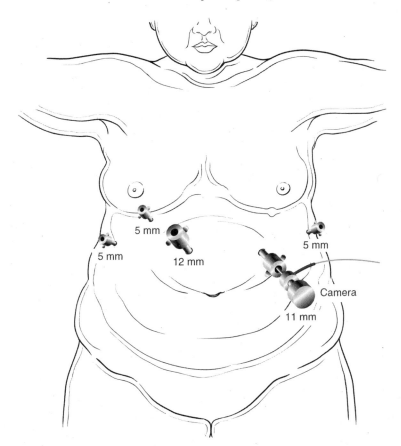

Figure 16.1. Trocar Position for laparoscopic staged Roux-en-Y.

9. The small bowel is clamped. An endoscopy is performed to test the integrity of the anastomosis with air insufflation while the anastomosis is submerged under water.

10. Close port sites larger than 5 mm at the fascial level.

E. Laparoscopic Staged Roux-en-Y (Second Stage)

1. The surgeon stands on the patient's right side. The assistant surgeon stands on the patient's left side.

2. An upper endoscopy is performed to examine for marginal ulceration. Place the endoscope through the gastrojejunal anastomosis.

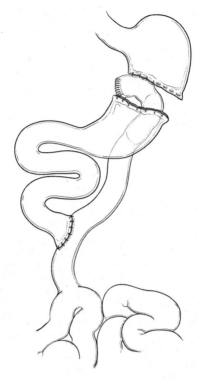

Figure 16.2. Laparoscopic staged Roux-en-Y (1st stage): Laparoscopic construction of a modified Roux-en-Y gastric bypass with a large gastric pouch and a low gastrojejunal anastomosis to minimize tension.

3. A laparoscopic exploration is performed with five abdominal trocars (see Fig. 16.1).
4. The gastrojejunal anastomosis is identified with the endoscope in place.
5. The gastric pouch is mobilized along the greater curvature using the ultrasonic shear.
6. A sleeve gastrectomy is performed (see Fig. 16.3), using multiple applications of the linear staplers (green load), starting at the level of the gastrojejunal anastomosis and completed at the Angle of His.
7. The endoscope is withdrawn and insufflated to check the integrity of the gastric pouch staple lines.
8. The sleeve gastrectomy specimen is removed through an enlarged trocar.

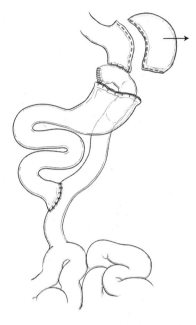

Figure 16.3. Laparoscopic staged Roux-en-Y (2nd stage): a sleeve gastrectomy is performed to reduce the volume of the gastric pouch.

F. Selected References

Nguyen NT, Longoria M, Gelfand DV, et al. Staged laparoscopic Roux-en-Y: a novel two-stage bariatric operation as an alternative in the super-obese with massively enlarged liver. Obes Surg 2005;15:1077–1081.

Oliak D, Ballantyne GH, Davies RJ, et al. Short-term results of laparoscopic gastric bypass in patients with BMI > or = 60. Obes Surg 2002;12:643–647.

Regan JP, Inabnet WB, Gagner M, et al. Early experience with two-stage laparoscopic Roux-en-Y gastric bypass as an alternative in the super-super obese patient. Obes Surg 2003;13:861–864.

III. Outcomes

17. Outcomes of Laparoscopic Gastric Bypass

Samuel Szomstein and Olga N. Tucker

A. Introduction

In the morbidly obese, surgery is the most effective option to achieve weight loss with resolution of comorbidity. Since its first description in 1967, the gastric bypass (RYGB) has continued to gain popularity. The introduction of the laparoscopic approach by Wittgrove in 1994 further increased patient acceptance, and it is now the most common bariatric procedure performed worldwide. The advantages of the laparoscopic approach include reduced mean operative time, operative blood loss, length of intensive care stay, postoperative pain, and in-hospital stay, with a faster recovery compared with the open technique with similar perioperative morbidity and mortality rates. The laparoscopic RYGB (LRYGB) procedure achieves weight loss by a combination of moderate restriction by reduction in gastric volume to 15 to 30 ml with a narrow outlet, the dumping syndrome in response to ingestion of food with a high sugar or fat content, and micronutrient malabsorption.

Short-term outcome after LRYGB is determined by surgical technique, surgeon volume, hospital volume, and surgical reintervention rate. Early outcome measures include perioperative rates of morbidity and mortality, surgical reintervention rate, and readmission rate. Early complications are classified as those occurring in the first 30 days after surgery, and late complications as those observed after 30 days. Major complications are life-threatening complications and/or those that lead to early reoperation. Long-term outcome is determined by the avoidance of nutritional deficiencies, early detection and treatment of complications, and close follow-up in a multidisciplinary care program.

B. Short-Term Outcome

1. Perioperative mortality

Operative mortality (<30 days) (0.2–1.9%).
 Risk factors:

- Body mass index
- Male gender

- Age
- Comorbidities

Cause:

- Anastomotic leak with sepsis
- Pulmonary embolus (0.2%)

2. Perioperative morbidity

Anastomotic leak:

- Incidence: 0.9–4.4%
- Staple line
- Gastrojejunal
- Jejunojejunal

Hemorrhage:

- Incidence: 1.1–3.8%
- Gastric pouch
- Gastric remnant
- Gastrojejunostomy
- Jejunojejunostomy
- Other source

Small bowel obstruction:

- Incidence: 0.6–3.8%
- Trocar site hernia
- Anastomotic stenosis or edema
  - ○ Gastrojejunal
  - ○ Jejunojejunal
- Intussusception
- Hematoma
  - ○ Intramural
  - ○ Intraluminal
  - ○ Mesenteric
- Internal hernia
  - ○ Incidence: 0.2–0.7%
  - ○ Petersen's space
  - ○ Mesocolic defect
  - ○ Jejunojejunostomy defect

Acute gastric remnant distention:
  Deep venous thrombosis
  Pulmonary embolus
  Abdominal compartment syndrome

Wound infection:

- Incidence: 0.1–8.7%
- Dehiscence

Rhabdomyolysis + acute renal failure

C. Long-Term Outcome

An appropriate follow-up program after LRYGB should detect:

- Weight loss
- Weight regain/failure to lose weight
- Comorbidity resolution
- Surgical complications
- Metabolic/nutritional complications
- Psychological stability
- Mortality

1. Weight loss

Mean percentage of excess weight loss (EWL%) 62% at 2 years (range 57–66%)

2. Weight regain/failure to lose weight

Weight regain
    5% regain weight at 12–13 months
    15% regain weight at 18 months to 2 years
    Cause:

- Errors in technique: large pouch, large stoma
- Binge eating
- Low energy expenditure

Failure to lose weight
    15% failure of weight loss at 3 years

3. Comorbidity resolution

Resolution of comorbid conditions:

- Diabetes: resolution in 77%
- Hyperlipidemia: improvement in 70%
- Hypertension: resolution in 62%
- Sleep apnea: resolution in 85%

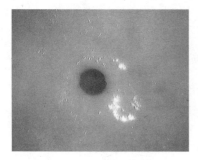 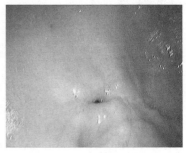

Figure 17.1. Upper gastrointestinal endoscopy after laparoscopic Roux-en-Y gastric bypass. **a.** Normal gastrojejunostomy. **b.** Stenosis of gastrojejunostomy.

4. Surgical complications

Chronic early:

- Marginal ulceration, hemorrhage, abdominal pain
- Small bowel obstruction: internal hernias, Petersen's defect, mesocolic defect, biliopancreatic limb
- Pouch dilatation
- Anastomotic (stomal) dilation (gastrojejunostomy) (Fig. 17.1)
- Anastomotic strictures: gastrojejunal (incidence: 1.6–11.4%), jejuno jejunal
- Biliary tract pathology: symptomatic gallstones, acute cholecystitis, choledocholithiasis
- Gastropathic fistulae (Fig. 17.2)

Chronic late:

- Weight regain
- Failure of weight loss
- Malnutrition

5. Metabolic/nutritional complications

Restriction of oral intake and malabsorption following LRYGB can result in nutritional deficiencies with metabolic consequences. Following LRYGB adequate oral intake with daily vitamin and mineral supplementation is essential with regular assessment by the dietician. Following LRYGB, pregnancy should be not considered for the first 18 months after surgery.

The following deficiencies may arise after LRYGB:

- Fat-soluble vitamins: A, D, E, K
- Water-soluble vitamins: B_1 thiamine, B_2 riboflavin, B_3 niacin, biotin, pantothenic acid, B_6, B_{12}, folic acid, C
- Minerals: iron, calcium, zinc

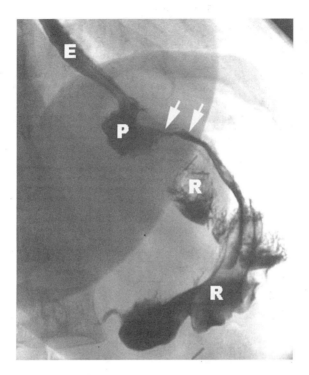

Figure 17.2. Gastrografin upper gastrointestinal contrast study demonstrating contrast extravasation from the gastric pouch (*P*) through a fistulous tract (*arrows*) into the remnant stomach (R). E = esophagus.

- Proteins
- Lipids
- Carbohydrates

A deficiency in carbohydrate absorption can augment protein or lipid deficiency as the body shifts toward gluconeogenesis.

6. Psychological stability

Deaths caused by suicide are 2.03 times as great after RYGB than in matched control patients.

7. Mortality

Long-term mortality (at 7.1 years):

- Death rate 2.7%
- Reduction in mortality from any cause, 40%

- Reduction in cause-specific mortality: coronary artery disease 56%; diabetes 92%; cancer 60%
- Estimated number of lives saved 136/100,000 gastric bypasses

D. Revisional Surgery

1. Revisional surgery for complications
   Indications:

   - Acute: technical problems/complications

     ○ Anastomotic leak
     ○ Bleeding
     ○ Gastric dilatation
     ○ Small bowel obstruction

   - Chronic: early (technical problems)

     ○ Anastomotic stricture
     ○ Anastomotic ulceration
     ○ Gastropathic fistula
     ○ Internal hernia
     ○ Slippage (banded gastroplasty)

   - Late: remedial/metabolic problems

     ○ Malnutrition
     ○ Weight regain
     ○ Failure of weight loss

2. Revisional surgery for debilitating morbidity
3. Revisional surgery for failed gastric bypass
   - Inadequate weight loss
   - Weight regain
   - Non resolution of comorbidity
   - Error in technique: Large pouch, large stoma

E. Selected References

Adams TD, Gress RE, Smith SC, et al. Long-term mortality after gastric bypass surgery. N Engl J Med 2007;357(8):753–761.

Buchwald H, Avidor Y, Braunwald E, et al. Bariatric surgery: a systematic review and meta-analysis. JAMA 2004;292(14):1724–1737.

Fernandez AZ, Jr., DeMaria EJ, Tichansky DS, et al. Multivariate analysis of risk factors for death following gastric bypass for treatment of morbid obesity. Ann Surg 2004;239(5):698–702.

Hall JC, Watts JM, O'Brien PE, et al. Gastric surgery for morbid obesity. The Adelaide Study. Ann Surg 1990;211(4):419–427.

Rosenthal RJ, Szomstein S, Kennedy CI, et al. Laparoscopic surgery for morbid obesity: 1,001 consecutive bariatric operations performed at The Bariatric Institute, Cleveland Clinic, Florida. Obes Surg 2006;16(2):119–124.

Wittgrove AC, Clark GW. Laparoscopic gastric bypass, Roux-en-Y- 500 patients: technique and results, with 3–60 month follow-up. Obes Surg 2000;10(3):233–239.

18. Outcomes of Laparoscopic Adjustable Gastric Banding

David A. Provost

A. Introduction

Laparoscopic adjustable gastric banding (LAGB) is a proven effective procedure for the treatment of morbid obesity. The most common bariatric procedure outside of the United States, LAGB has increased rapidly in the United States since its introduction in 2001. Touted advantages of LAGB over Roux-en-Y gastric bypass (RYGB) include its technically simpler laparoscopic approach, reduced perioperative morbidity, and mortality, adjustability, and reversibility. Numerous studies from Europe and Australia had documented significant and durable weight loss with improvement or resolution of associated comorbidities following LAGB placement with follow-up beyond 5 years, and contemporary reports from the United States parallel international results.

Despite favorable outcomes with LAGB in most recent publications, disappointing results with LAGB continue to be reported in some series, with high rates of reoperation, band loss, and poor weight loss. Two factors account for these conflicting results. The replacement of perigastric dissection with the *pars flaccida* technique for band placement has dramatically decreased the rate of complications and band extirpations. Weight loss is dependent upon postoperative follow-up and appropriate band adjustments. Frequent, clinically based adjustments are necessary to maintain the proper degree of restriction and successful weight loss. LAGB placement using the pars flaccida technique, combined with appropriate adjustment schedules and follow-up are mandatory for optimal outcomes.

B. Perioperative Outcomes

A major advantage of the LAGB is its safety. An evidence-based review by the Australian Safety and Efficacy Register of New Interventional Procedures-Surgical ASERNIP-S) found that LAGB was associated with a median overall morbidity rate of 11.3% with a mean short-term mortality of 0.05%. This compares with 23.6% morbidity and 0.5% mortality for RYGB. In 14 series from the United States utilizing the *pars flaccida* technique, overall operative mortality was 0.08%. Gastric or esophageal perforation during band placement is reported in 0% to 0.4%, venous thromboembolism in 0.1% to 0.2%, and wound infections in 1%. Open conversion is required in less than 1% of cases.

Early obstruction, a problem reported in 1% to 8% of early series using the pars flaccida technique, has virtually been eliminated with the introduction of larger-diameter bands and recognition of the importance of excising excessive perigastric fat when the band appears tight.

C. Late Complications

Late band-related complications plagued early series of LAGB, with prolapse rates of 15% to 40% and extirpation rates as high as 60% when using the perigastric technique. Port and tubing complications requiring reoperation occurred in 10% to 20%, until the introduction of a redesigned port and refined placement techniques.

Studies utilizing the perigastric technique are of historical interest only. Contemporary results with the *pars flaccida* technique yield prolapse rates less than 5%, erosions in fewer than 1%, port related complications in 2% to 6%, and band extirpations in fewer than 3% of patients undergoing LAGB. Esophageal dilatation and esophageal reflux occur only with over-tightening of the band, responding to fluid removal, or with prolapse, and is reported infrequently. Symptoms of reflux following LAGB should lead to prompt loosening of the band and investigation of band position. When care is taken, esophageal dilation is an avoidable complication.

D. Weight Loss

Weight loss following LAGB is clearly dependent upon proper band adjustments and a frequent adjustment schedule during the first 1 to 2 years postoperatively. The need for frequent adjustments results from the loss of perigastric fat within the band with weight loss, loosening the band, and permitting increased intake. Weight loss following LAGB is significantly slower than following RYGB, so comparisons between the operations demonstrate superior weight loss for RYGB when early results are reported. Weight loss continues beyond 3 to 4 years in most series, and late regain has been infrequently reported. Potential benefits of the gradual weight loss observed with LAGB include a reduced incidence of nutritional deficiencies, hair loss, and cholelithiasis. With follow-up of 4 to 9 years, percent excess weight loss exceeds 50% in the majority of series, comparing favorably with the long-term weight loss reported after RYGB.

The need for appropriate follow-up and adjustment with LAGB cannot be overemphasized. Shen et al. demonstrated that weight loss with LAGB is related to the frequency of follow-up, in contrast to RYGB. Regularly scheduled visits, at 4- to 6-week intervals for the first year or two postoperatively, with adjustments as needed, will produce optimal results. Patients who fail to return for follow-up visits are more likely to have poorer results.

E. Comorbidity Resolution

Weight loss is a benefit of bariatric surgery, but improvements in comorbid illness and quality of life are the primary goals. Type 2 diabetes mellitus is a major contributor to the long-term morbidity associated with morbid obesity. While the immediate impact on insulin resistance observed following RYGB is not seen with LAGB, with weight loss improvement or resolution of diabetes in 65% to 80% of patients is observed after LAGB. Hypertension resolves or improves in 60% to 85%. LAGB has also been demonstrated to improve lipid profiles, asthma, sleep apnea, menstrual irregularities and infertility, depression, joint and back pain, stress incontinence, self-esteem, and overall quality of life.

Early reports of an increased rate of gastroesophageal reflux (GERD) following LAGB and an increased incidence of prolapse in patients with hiatal hernia have led some to question LAGB placement in the presence of a hiatal hernia. Reflux following LAGB is usually an indication of an overly tightened band or a sign of prolapse or pouch dilatation, a complication greatly reduced by the adoption of the *pars flaccida* approach. O'Brien reported total resolution of GERD in 89% of LAGB patients, improvement in 5%, no change in 2.5%, and aggravation of symptoms in 2.5%.

F. Conclusions

LAGB provides a safer option for morbidly obese patients seeking weight loss, with an incidence of complications one half of the rate following gastric bypass, and one tenth the mortality. Complications, unlike anastamotic leaks or intestinal obstruction, are rarely life threatening but must be balanced against the risk of erosion and increased need for revision. Most importantly, weight loss has proved durable. Laparoscopic adjustable gastric banding is a safe and effective option for the morbidly obese patient seeking weight loss surgery.

G. Selected References

Chapman AE, Kiroff G, Game P, et al. Laparoscopic adjustable gastric banding in the treatment of obesity: a systematic literature review. Surgery 2004;135(3):326–351.

O'Brien PE, Dixon JD, et al. A prospective randomized trial of placement of the laparoscopic adjustable gastric band: comparison of the perigastric and pars flaccida pathways. Obes Surg 2005;15:820–826.

Ponce J, Paynter S, Fromm R. Laparoscopic adjustable gastric banding: 1,014 consecutive cases. J Am Coll Surg 2005;201:529–535.

Shen R, Dugay G, Rajaram K, et al. Impact of patient follow-up on weight loss after bariatric surgery. Obes Surg 2004;14:514–519.

19. Outcomes of Duodenal Switch and Other Malabsorptive Procedures

Peter F. Crookes

A. Background

The first bariatric operations were entirely malabsorptive and left the stomach untouched. They came to be known as jejunoileal bypass (JIB). In the most popular version of JIB, the jejunum was divided 14 inches beyond the ligament of Treitz and the proximal end anastomosed to the terminal ileum 4 inches from the ileocecal valve (the 14-4 operation). The stimulus to their development was derived from recognition of the short gut syndrome, in which it was clear that patients with massive intestinal resection lost weight despite a high oral intake. The first formal program to follow a series of obese patients after intestinal bypass was developed by a private practice surgeon (J. Howard Payne) and an endocrinologist (Loren DeWind) in Los Angeles, beginning in 1957. Their careful reports identified a number of serious complications that could make their appearance many years after the surgery. These complications included protein-calorie malnutrition and vitamin deficiencies, electrolyte imbalance, renal calculi, and local perianal problems, as a consequence of the extreme malabsorption and the diarrhea it produced. Further, arthropathy and progressive liver failure occurred in a significant percentage of patients, evidently the result of bacterial overgrowth in the lengthy blind loop of intestine (all but 45 cm). Despite the beneficial effects of weight loss and resolution of major comorbidities such as diabetes mellitus, hyperlipidemia, and obstructive sleep apnea, the frequency and potential severity of these problems, often requiring reversal of the bypass, led to the abandonment of intestinal bypass in favor of purely restrictive procedures or a Roux-en-Y reconstruction to a small gastric pouch.

These disadvantages prompted the Italian surgeon Nicola Scopinaro to develop a malabsorptive procedure in which the degree of malabsorption was more controlled and the blind limb of proximal intestine was exposed to bile and pancreatic juice, thus avoiding the problems of bacterial overgrowth in the defunctionalized small bowel. This operation, termed biliopancreatic diversion (BPD), thus avoided most of the complications of the original JIB. Scopinaro has the longest follow-up of any bariatric surgeon and recently reported results with a mean of 18-year follow-up. The characteristics of the BPD are illustrated in Fig. 19.1. In brief, a distal gastrectomy involving all the antrum and some of the body of the stomach is performed, leaving a pouch estimated at 200 to 500 ml capacity. The small bowel is divided 250 cm from the ileocecal valve, and the proximal end

158   P F Crookes

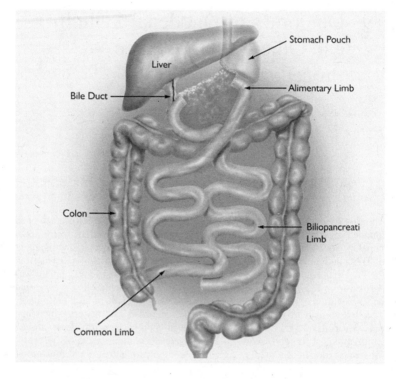

Figure 19.1. Schematic representation of biliopancreatic diversion procedure.

(biliopancreatic limb) anastomosed to the ileum 50 cm from the ileocecal valve. The distal end of the transected bowel (alimentary limb, or Roux limb) is anastomosed to the gastric pouch. The logic behind the operation is that the restriction of the stomach is minimal, allowing essentially unrestricted eating: carbohydrate and some protein absorption is possible in the alimentary limb, but fat absorption is restricted to the short common channel since it requires the presence of bile and pancreatic enzymes. This accounts for the relatively selective fat malabsorption induced by the BPD, as well as the beneficial effect on lipid and cholesterol metabolism.

The BPD appears to be less popular outside Italy, because of the perceived risk of various types of malnutrition. This led the Spanish surgeon Alvaro Larrad-Jimenez to propose a modification in which the biliopancreatic limb is limited to 50 cm, the common channel to 50 cm, and the alimentary limb the remainder. This operation, termed the 50-50 BPD, is claimed to produce comparable weight loss but with less severe nutritional complications.

However, the modification of the BPD most widely adopted has been the procedure commonly termed the duodenal switch (DS), developed by Marceau et al. in Quebec and Hess et al. in the United States. It differs from the BPD in that the stomach remnant is not a proximal stomach pouch, but a narrow gastric tube based on the lesser curve, preserving the distal antrum and pylorus, with the alimentary limb being anastomosed to the end of the first part of the duodenum (Fig. 19.2). Because it is more restrictive than the BPD, the degree of malabsorption is made less extreme, with a common channel usually 75 to 100 cm or more. The operation is technically more complex than BPD because of the difficulty of the dissection of the second part of the duodenum. It is also considerably more difficult to perform laparoscopically. This chapter summarizes the outcome of these malabsorptive procedures and expresses outcome in the context of the most widely performed bariatric procedure, namely the Roux-en-Y gastric bypass (RNY GBP). It must be emphasized at the outset that Level 1 evidence within the bariatric literature is very rare. The majority of published reports are of uncontrolled studies with incomplete and short follow-up intervals. Nevertheless, this is what is available, and understanding the limitations of such reports is the best way to assess the outcome of a given procedure.

B. Outcomes

Outcome measures are generally cited by reporting the effect of surgery on: (a) weight loss, (b) resolution of comorbidities, and (c) quality of life. Complications and other unwanted effects are the subject of another chapter and

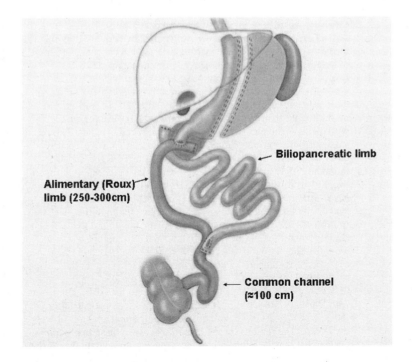

Figure 19.2. Schematic representation of duodenal switch procedure.

will be briefly summarized here. All outcome measures are difficult to compare because of differences in the duration and completeness of follow-up in individual reports. The most comprehensive published summary is the meta-analysis of Buchwald et al. (2004) where outcomes of a total of 22,094 patients were categorized. From this paper it is clear that BPD with or without DS has comparable weight loss to gastric bypass.

1. Weight loss

a. Pathophysiology of weight loss. It is often asserted that DS is a purely malabsorptive operation. This is incorrect: In contrast to the BPD, in which the reservoir portion of the stomach is essentially untouched, the DS procedure involves a substantial gastric resection leaving the stomach as a fairly narrow tube based on the lesser curve. The anatomy of the lesser curve is characterized by tough horizontal "clasp" fibers, and the amount of stomach that can respond to food ingestion by receptive relaxation is very limited. Therefore, it combines a substantial amount of restriction. Many surgeons who perform sleeve gastrectomy as a stand-alone procedure make the stomach narrower (using a smaller indwelling bougie) than if it is being performed as part of a DS. However, in the early weeks after DS, food capacity is not much more than that experienced by GBP patients. We studied the patients' perception of their food intake after weight stabilization and reported that they can eat an estimated 30% to 50% of their preoperative intake.

Loss of appetite and early satiety are reported by patients after DS. The underlying pathophysiologic mechanisms are still obscure, but removal of the fundus and reduction of ghrelin secretion may play a part.

b. Degree of weight loss after BPD and DS. Within the bariatric community, and especially among patients who express their views on websites, there is a strong belief that weight loss after DS is both greater and more durable than after RNY GBP procedures. There are few rigorous studies in the published literature to support this belief. Two recent studies from respected centers in Portland and Chicago each reported head-to-head non-randomized comparisons of RNY and DS: One found no difference in weight loss, whereas the other reported superior weight loss in superobese patients (BMI >50) after DS compared with RNY GBP. In both studies, there was a tendency to perform DS for the heavier patients with more severe metabolic abnormalities. The study from Portland followed patients for 2 years, and found that DS had a slightly longer length of hospital stay, a slightly higher leak rate, but mortality was similar (0.8% for GBP vs. 0.9% for DS), and EBWL was 67% for GBP compared with 63% for DS after 2 years. In the Chicago study length of stay was also slightly longer for DS vs. GBP, mortality was low in both groups (0.05% for DS, zero for GBP), but patients with DS tended to have greater EBWL (72%) than patients after GBP (60%) after 2 years, with both groups gaining small amounts of weight by 3 years. The reasons for the disparity between these two studies are unclear, but may be a function of incomplete follow-up. In the Portland study only 93 of the original 350 patients were available for follow-up 2 years later, and in the Chicago study, also with 350 patients, only 65 had 3-year follow-up. In light of this incomplete evidence, it would appear that DS or BPD does not have a reliable superiority over RNY GBP except possibly in the superobese.

2. Relief of comorbidities

Some of the typical comorbidities are primarily a function of physically increased weight, and only improve as weight loss occurs. Degenerative joint disease in the spine and weight-bearing joints, urinary incontinence, obstructive sleep apnea, and pulmonary impairment are in this category. Other problems, such as diabetes, dyslipidemia, and possibly hypertension are related to altered metabolism and may improve even before any weight loss occurs. Different procedures thus have different effects on these metabolically -induced comorbidities. Purely restrictive procedures, although partially effective in resolving diabetes and dyslipidemia, are less effective than bypass procedures such as RNY, GBP, and BPD/DS.

a.   Type 2 diabetes. Relief of diabetes after BPD and DS appears to be greater than with any other operation. In the meta-analysis of Buchwald, 17 studies involving 4,096 patients were analyzed, with improvement or resolution noted in 98%, higher than after any other procedure analyzed in this study. The recent work of Rubino and colleagues has identified two major mechanisms whereby glucose tolerance is improved after bariatric surgery, which may be summarized as a proximal gut factor and a distal gut factor. The proximal factor is related to the diversion of food away from the duodenum, through mechanisms as yet unidentified, appears to improve glucose control. This proximal mechanism is operative in BPD, DS, and RNYGBP, but not after purely restrictive procedures such as the lap-band or sleeve gastrectomy. The distal factor appears to result from undigested food reaching the ileum, and is believed to be mediated by the release of GLP-1. GLP-1 delays gastric emptying and enhances insulin secretion and stimulates the formation of more β-cells in the pancreatic islets. This distal mechanism is more pronounced in malabsorptive operations such as BPD and DS and results in superior resolution of diabetes and impaired glucose tolerance compared with any other bariatric procedure.

c.   Hyperlipidemia. For similar reasons, the distal fat-malabsorbing effect of BPD and DS cause almost universal reduction of cholesterol and triglycerides, in the few studies in which these measurements were made.

d.   Obstructive sleep apnea. Unlike diabetes and dyslipidemias, improvement in sleep apnea is dependent on weight loss, and in published reports averages 80% to 90%, which is not significantly different from the degree of improvement in other contemporary operations.

e.   Weight-related comorbidities. Many of these conditions such as degenerative joint disease and urinary stress incontinence are not easily quantified. Many morbidly obese patients who would otherwise be good candidates for joint replacement surgery are recommended to lose weight before such surgery will be considered. We recently reported that the long-term outcome of knee replacement was not affected by moderate degrees of obesity, offering some reassurance that patients whose weight is reduced to a BMI in the region of 30 kg/m^2 can undergo joint replacement without sabotaging the operation.

Improvement in musculoskeletal conditions, especially involving the spine, foot, and ankle, were recently reported for gastric bypass, in which the percentage of patients reporting such symptoms dropped from 100% to 37% after surgery. However, comparable studies have not been reported for BPD or DS.

f. What is the cost? Long-term side effects and problems after BPD and DS. Despite the beneficial effects achieved by these procedures, there remains worry that long-term problems of malnutrition may detract from the early benefits.

Almost all patients who achieve sufficient weight loss report increased malodorous flatulence and more frequent bowel movements. These symptoms tend to be related to fat intake, and may be associated with crampy abdominal pain. As patients learn how the reconstructed intestinal tract responds to different foods, some adaptation takes place. Dumping in response to sweet intake tends to be rare. Although intuitively it was suggested that the preservation of the pylorus in the DS led to improved symptomatic outcome compared with BPD, the only study to compare the symptomatic outcome of the two procedures detected no differences between them.

g. Long-term deficiencies. All patients after any kind of bypass, whether GBP or DS, have a problem with Iron and calcium absorption, since both are normally absorbed in the bypassed portion of the GI tract. Consequently, microcytic anemia is common, especially in younger women who are still menstruating. Even before the serum iron is abnormal, defective iron stores are detectable when serum ferritin drops and the total iron-binding capacity increases. Oral supplementation with ferrous sulfate is the cheapest and most readily available method, but ferrous gluconate or fumarate may be more easily absorbed. If iron levels are persistently subnormal despite oral supplements, a loading dose of intravenous iron may be given, usually under the supervision of a hematologist.

Macrocytic anemia is rarely seen after BPD and DS, since it is not common for B$_{12}$ and folate levels to be low unless patients fail to comply with the prescribed vitamin supplementation regimen. As a class, DS patients tend to be knowledgeable and motivated; hence, this is rarely a problem.

Calcium deficiency may not be immediately apparent, because serum calcium tends to remain in the low normal range. Indirect evidence of defective calcium absorption may be sought by measuring parathyroid hormone (PTH). We recently reported that elevated PTH was more common in patients after DS with 75 cm common channel compared with those in whom the common channel was 100 cm long. Vitamin D levels tend to be lower after DS because vitamin D is a fat-soluble vitamin and is poorly absorbed. The best estimate of vitamin D stores is 25 (OH) D. In contrast, levels of 1,25 (OH)2 D are increased by PTH in the presence of vitamin D deficiency. Vitamin D is important in promoting absorption of calcium from the gut, but it also has independent effects on muscle strength and patients with vitamin D deficiency frequently report weakness, tiredness, and fatigability, which is then labeled with diagnoses such as fibromyalgia and chronic fatigue syndrome. Even after aggressive oral supplementation of vitamin D, absorption may still be inadequate. The easiest way to enhance vitamin D is solar exposure, especially in white individuals. When this is not possible, twice weekly intramuscular injections of vitamin D may be given for a period of several weeks until stores are repleted.

Clinical vitamin A deficiency is rarely reported in isolation, but it has been reported in the ophthalmology literature. Since it is a fat soluble vitamin it may be malabsorbed in the same way as vitamin D. The major effects of vitamin A deficiency are ocular.

Protein-calorie malnutrition is characterized by muscle loss, excessive weight loss, hypoalbuminemia, and frequently edema. Unlike the malnutrition associated with poor intake, it is often associated with diarrhea, and hypokalemia.

All of the preceding deficiencies were more frequent when short common channels (50 cm) were employed. In our experience and that of others, a common channel of 100 cm is associated with a reduced incidence of such problems. The incidence of malnutrition of such severity as to require partial revision of the operation varies from 2% to 5%. The most common scenario is a combination of excessive weight loss with edema and diarrhea. The simplest way to correct the degree of malabsorption is to perform a side-to-side anastomosis between the biliopancreatic and alimentary limbs (the "kissing X anastomosis"). Weight regain is surprisingly limited after this procedure, averaging about 15 lbs, and there is good correction of albumin, hemoglobin, and potassium.

h. Other late outcomes BPD and DS, like other bypass procedures, have an intrinsic proclivity to lead to small bowel obstruction, often many years afterward. This may be due to internal herniation, simple adhesions, or kinking at the jejunojejunostomy. A unique form of obstruction after BPD and DS can be caused by obstruction of the biliopancreatic limb. Small case series of this important complication have been reported, but the denominator is not known and therefore assessment of the risk is imprecise. The biliopancreatic limb in BPD and DS is long, approximately 300 cm, and it ends blindly at the second portion of the duodenum. Therefore, it acts like other forms of closed loop obstruction, and the development of ischemia and gangrene is rapid. It cannot be decompressed by NG suction, it is inaccessible to endoscopy, and since the alimentary limb often remains open, the other typical features of small bowel obstruction are not present. All patients presenting with severe crampy abdominal pain persisting for more than a few hours should seek urgent medical attention and undergo CT scanning, since this is the only way to make the diagnosis quickly (Fig. 19.3). Since the patient may present to another hospital where the DS is not performed, the general surgeon on call may be unfamiliar with the anatomical alterations of BPD or DS procedures, and may waste valuable time in attempting to transfer the patient to the original operating surgeon.

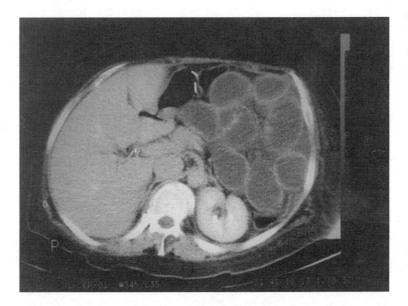

Figure 19.3. Abdominal CT Scan showing biliopancreatic obstruction. Note the distended loops without contrast.

Patients with the BPD and DS should be given a card with a diagram or other depiction of their reconstruction, and should be warned to seek help for persistent (>6 hours) abdominal pain.

i.   Special situations. Pregnancy after BPD and DS is generally uneventful. However, there is more concern over vitamin deficiencies, and patients of childbearing age must be especially counseled to maintain compliance with vitamin and mineral supplements. Isolated cases of microphthalmia, caused by vitamin A deficiency at the critical stage of organogenesis, have been reported, but there is no systematic study of pregnancy after BPD or DS.

C. Selected References

Anthone GJ, Lord RV, DeMeester TR, et al. The duodenal switch operation for the treatment of morbid obesity. Ann Surg 2003;238:618–628.

Buchwald H, Avidor Y, Braunwald E, et al. Bariatric surgery: a systematic review and meta-analysis. JAMA 2004;292(14):1724–1737.

Cossu ML, Meloni GB, Alagna S, et al. Emergency surgical conditions after biliopancreatic diversion. Obes Surg 2007;17(5):637–641.

Deveney CW, MacCabee D, Marlink K, et al. Roux-en-Y divided gastric bypass results in the same weight loss as duodenal switch for morbid obesity. Am J Surg 2004;187:655–659.

Dolan K, Hatzifotis M, Newbury L, et al. A clinical and nutritional comparison of biliopancreatic diversion with and without duodenal switch. Ann Surg 2004;240:51–56.

Hamoui N, Cantor S, Anthone GJ, et al. Effect of obesity on long term outcome of total knee arthroplasty. Obes Surg 2006;16:35–38.

Hamoui N, Chock B, Anthone GJ, et al. Revision of the duodenal switch: technique, indications, and outcome. J Am Coll Surg 2007;204(4):603–608.

Hamoui N, Kim K, Anthone G, et al. The significance of elevated levels of parathyroid hormone in patients with morbid obesity before and after bariatric surgery. Arch Surg 2003;138:891–897.

Hess DS, Hess DW, Oakley RS. The biliopancreatic diversion with the duodenal switch: results beyond 10 years. Obes Surg 2005;15:408–416.

Hooper MM, Stellato TA, Hallowell PT, et al. Musculoskeletal findings in obese subjects before and after weight loss following bariatric surgery. Int J Obes (Lond) 2007;31(1):114–1120.

Larrad-Jimenez A, Diaz-Guerra CS, de Cuadros Borrajo P, et al. Short-, mid- and long-term results of Larrad biliopancreatic diversion. Obes Surg 2007;17:202–210.

Marceau P, Biron S, Bourque RA, et al. Biliopancreatic diversion with a new type of gastrectomy. Obes Surg 1993;3:29–35.

Marceau P, Hould FS, Simard S, et al. Biliopancreatic diversion with duodenal switch. World J Surg 1998;22:947–954.

Polizzi A, Schenone M, Sacca SC, et al. Role of impression cytology during hypovitaminosis A. Br J Ophthalmol 1998;82(3):303–305.

Prachand VN, Davee RT, Alverdy JC. Duodenal switch provides superior weight loss in the super-obese (BMI > or = 50 kg/m^2) compared with gastric bypass. Ann Surg 2006;244(4):611–619.

Rubino F, Forgione A, Cummings DE, et al. The mechanism of diabetes control after gastrointestinal bypass surgery reveals a role of the proximal small intestine in the pathophysiology of type 2 diabetes. Ann Surg 2006;244(5):741–749.

Scopinaro N. Biliopancreatic diversion: mechanisms of action and long-term results. Obes Surg 2006;16(6):683–689.

Scopinaro N, Adami GF, Marinari GM, et al. Biliopancreatic diversion. World J Surg 1998;22(9):936–946.

Smets KJ, Barlow T, Vanhaesebrouck P. Maternal vitamin A deficiency and neonatal microphthalmia: complications of biliopancreatic diversion? Eur J Pediatr 2006;165(7):502–504.

20. Outcomes of Bariatric Surgery in Adolescents

Go Miyano and Thomas H. Inge

A. Epidemiologic Trends and Behavioral Weight Management

The adult obesity epidemic has grown in severity over the past several decades, and an equally worrisome rise in obesity prevalence in children ominously portends a future worsening of this obesity epidemic in all ages. The prevalence of adolescent obesity has tripled over the last three decades and approximately 4% of US children are currently affected with extreme obesity (BMI for age >99th percentile). The consequences of pediatric and adolescent obesity are becoming clearer, and are worrisome.

Although it is widely held that behavioral and dietary treatment approaches have greater efficacy for pediatric obesity than for adult obesity, extreme pediatric obesity is usually not amenable to either conventional dietary and medication regimens, with only a 2% to 3% decrease in BMI expected. Thus, it is unlikely that dietary interventions alone will effect durable long-term weight reduction and comorbidity resolution for most adolescents.

B. Surgical Weight Loss in Adolescents

Although numerous studies have now reported surgical outcomes for adolescents undergoing bariatric procedures, most report short-term outcomes with very limited follow-up, and all are retrospective in design. We examined the data from 13 recently published studies, seven of which reported outcomes after laparoscopic adjustable gastric banding (LAGB), and six of which reported outcomes after Roux-en-Y gastric bypass (RYGB).

1. BMI change after LAGB

Seven LAGB studies reported weight and BMI change, with length of follow-up ranging from 1.7 to 3.3 years. Study characteristics and weight and BMI data appear in Table 20.1 and Fig. 20.1. Among five larger case series, a total of 262 adolescent patients aged 9 to 19 were included, with an average mean preoperative BMI of 42 to 48 kg/m². The patients lost 37% to 70% of excess body weight during 6-month to 7-year follow-up. Long-term weight loss outcomes for the LAGB and standardized descriptions of comorbidity change are still lacking.

168   G Miyano and T H Inge

Table 20.1. Weight loss outcomes for LAGB and RYGB.

	n	*age*	*f/u (year)*	*BMI* pre-op	post-op	*%EWL*
LAGB						
Nadler (2007)	53	15.9		47.6		37.5–62.7
Yitzhak (2006)	60	16	3.3	43	30	
Silberhumer (2006)	50	17.1	2.9	45.2	32.6	61.4
Angrisani (2005)	58	18	3	46.1	37.8	39.7–55.6
Fielding (2005)	41	15.6	1.7	42.4	30.2	70
Horgan (2005)	4	17.8		50.5		15.0–87.0
Abu-Abeid (2003)	11	15.7	1.9	46.6	32.5	
RYGB						
Collins (2007)	11	16.5	1.8	50.5	28	60.8
Lawson (2006)	35	17.6	1	56.5	35.8	
Barnett (2005)	14	15.7		51		64
Sugerman (2003)	33	16	5	52	33	
Strauss (2001)	10	16.2	6.3	53.6	35.2	65
Rand (1994)	34	17	6	47	32	66

EWL: excess weight loss.

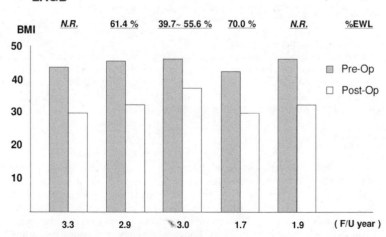

Figure 20.1. BMI before and after LAGB.

However, Yitzhak et al. reported that at least 80% of adolescents had sustained weight loss 5 years after AGB, and Fielding et al. reported 30% weight reduction 3 years postoperatively in 18 patients.

2. BMI change in the RYGB

Six studies reported weight and BMI data following RYGB with length of follow-up ranging from 1.0 to 6.3 years. Study characteristics and weight and BMI data appear in Table 20.1 and Fig. 20.2.

Lawson's study from Cincinnati Children's Hospital was a cohort-controlled multicenter study in which laparoscopic RYGB was compared with outcomes of extremely obese adolescents who participated for 1 year in a pediatric behavioral treatment program. Laparoscopic RYGB resulted in a change in mean BMI from 56.5 to 35.8 kg/m², as compared with no significant change in BMI in the comparison group with behavioral intervention. Strauss et al., evaluating results of gastric bypass in 10 adolescents, reported that mean preoperative BMI was 52.4 and maximal weight loss was achieved at 12 to 15 months postoperatively. Sugerman et al. have provided the largest retrospective study of adolescent bariatric surgery with the longest follow-up to date. Over a 21-year period, mean BMI measured preoperatively and at 1, 5, 10, and 14 years after surgery was 52, 36, 33, 34, and 38 kg/m², respectively. Five patients (15%) regained all or most of their lost weight at 5 to 10

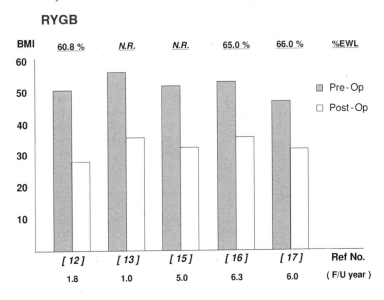

Figure 20.2. BMI before and after RYGB.

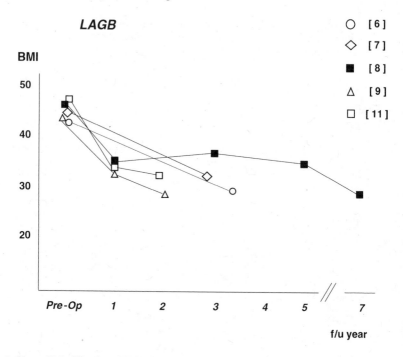

Figure 20.3. Kinetics of BMI change over time following LAGB.

years after surgery. The precise frequency of weight regain after adolescent RYGB is not clear, but is estimated to range from 10% to 20%. The postoperative BMI transition in both LAGB and RYGB is displayed graphically in Figs. 20.3 and 20.4.

C. Comorbidity

Five of seven LAGB studies reported comorbidity change, and the resolution rates were: 89% (8/9) for type 2 diabetes mellitus (T2DM), 100% (11/11) for obstructive sleep apnea syndrome (OSAS), and 65% (11/17) for hypertension (HTN). Four of six RYGB studies reported comorbidity data, the resolution rates were: 63% (5/8) for DM, 90% (18/20) for OSAS, and 75% (15/20) for HTN. A summary of the data appears in Table 20.1 and Fig. 20.5. These studies also in general reported favorable change in dyslipidemia, nonalcoholic steatohepatitis, gastroesophageal reflux disease, weight-related arthropathies, and pseudotumor cerebri, although it is important to consider the following limitation: These data are derived from very few published studies, often without clear documentation of how comorbidities were assessed preoperatively and postoperatively. These facts significantly limit our ability to accurately interpret or generalize from the findings.

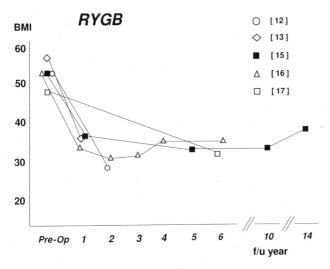

Figure 20.4. Kinetics of BMI change over time following RYGB.

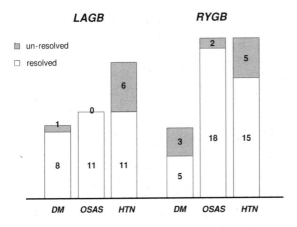

DM: Type 2 diabetic mellitus; OSAS: obstructive sleep apnea syndrome; HTN: hypertension.

Figure 20.5. Comorbidity change after adolescent bariatric surgery.

1. Type 2 diabetes mellitus

The most compelling reasons for performing bariatric procedures in adolescence are to reduce or resolve obesity-related comorbidity, and some of the most severe consequences of obesity seen in adolescents include T2DM and OSAS. A steep rise in prevalence of type 2 diabetes is occurring worldwide in parallel with an increasing rate of obesity in children and adolescents. When considering all of the as yet limited surgical outcome data (LAGB and RYGB studies), T2DM appears to resolve in 76% (13/17). In the adult surgical literature, duration of diabetes seems to predict completeness of resolution postoperatively. This may be an important factor when considering the timing of bariatric surgery for younger diabetic patients.

2. Obstructive sleep apnea syndrome

Marcus et al. reported abnormal polysomnograms in 36% of obese children and adolescents, and also showed a positive correlation between the degree of obesity and the severity of OSAS. When considering all available pediatric outcome data, OSAS resolution following LAGB and RYGB was 94% (29/31). Kalra et al., utilizing pre- and postoperative polysomnography, reported that OSAS was diagnosed in 55% of 34 patients studied preoperatively. Ten of these patients returned for follow-up PSG, and OSA significantly improved or resolved after RYGB in all the ten subjects, with nine of ten returning to a normal frequency of OSAS events.

3. Quality of life

Adverse psychosocial and educational consequences of extreme adolescent obesity are a topic of considerable concern, and being an overweight young adult has a lasting impact on life satisfaction and aspirations. Some have noted an increase in employment and educational status in those adolescents who lost the most weight postoperatively. Several recent studies also showed significant improvement in postoperative QOL after LAGB and RYGB in adolescents using formal measures.

D. Mortality and Postoperative Adverse Events

1. Mortality

No perioperative death was reported in both the LAGB and the RYGB. However, four late deaths not linked to the surgery or weight loss have been reported by Lawson, Barnett, and Sugarman.

2. The adverse events on the LAGB

All LAGB studies reported adverse events (summarized in Table 20.2). Twenty-six reoperations were performed to correct various complications in

Table 20.2. Adverse events after adolescent bariatric surgery.

	Comorbidity*			Mort	Adverse Event				
	DM	OSAS	HTN	(late death)	bs	def	ulc	dum	obs
LAGB									
Nadler (2007)				2	4				
Yitzhak (2006)	2	10	3	8					
Silber humer (2006)	5		12						
Angrisani (2005)	2		2	1					
Fielding (2005)		1		1					
Horgan (2005)									
Abu-Abeid (2003)						4			
RYGB									
Collins (2007)	6	2	6				2		
Lawson (2006)		10		1		4		1	
Barnett (2005)			11	1				2	
Sugerman (2003)	2	6	3	2			4		1
Strauss (2001)		2				8			1
Rand (1994)									

DM: Type 2 diabetic mellitus; OSAS: obstructive sleep apnea syndrome; HTN: hypertension; bs: band slippage; def: nutritional deficiency; dum: dumping syndrome; obs: gastrointestinal obstruction; ulc: marginal ulcer.
*Comorbidity: number of total cases (number of resolved cases).

the LAGB group, for an overall reoperation rate of 9%. Reasons for reoperation included band slippage, intragastric migration, and port/tubing problems. Band slippage was the most frequently reported post-LAGB complication, which occurred on 12 of the 277 patients (4.3%).

3. The adverse events on the RYGB

All six RYGB studies also reported adverse events (summarized in Table 20.2). Early complications of RYGB in adolescents included pulmonary embolism, postoperative bleeding, staple line leak, wound infection, stomal stenosis, and marginal ulceration. Late complications included small bowel obstruction, incisional hernias, severe malnutrition, symptomatic cholelithiasis, and late weight regain. Problems related to protein calorie malnutrition and micronutrient deficiency, such as iron, vitamin B_{12}, vitamin D, thiamine, and calcium, were the most frequently reported complications after RYGB. Since it is not known to what degree risks may increase over time, prospective long-term studies are vital to determine the true prevalence and clinical significance of complications, including mechanical/technical problems and nutritional deficiencies following bariatric surgery in adolescents.

E. Which Operation Is Best for Adolescents?

When gastric bypass and adjustable gastric banding have been compared, reports have cited greater weight loss and comorbidity resolution with gastric bypass at early time intervals (1–3 years), but similar weight loss efficacy at later time intervals (5 year). The appeal of adjustable gastric banding for adolescents lies in the reversibility, low incidence of morbidity and mortality, and potential avoidance of severe nutritional risks associated with malabsorptive procedures; however, potential worrisome later complications, including band obstruction, gastric prolapse, tubing problems, frequency of band explanation, will be critical for clinical decision making for adolescents who have perhaps five or six decades to live with the device. Although this device holds a great deal of promise for treatment of adolescent with extreme obesity, more information about long-term efficacy and durability is needed.

While biliopancreatic diversion (BPD) has been reported in adolescents, most believe that the risks of BPD and even duodenal switch likely outweigh their potential benefit of greater weight loss as compared with RYGB and AGB. For this reason, these operations are not recommended for most adolescents.

The laparoscopic sleeve gastrectomy (LSG) is a new operation that produces significant initial weight loss with low operative risk in adult studies. The LSG may be a safe option for adolescents with fewer nutritional and long-term device-related risks than other operations. However, further studies are needed to determine objectively the risk–benefit ratio for adolescents.

F. Selected References

Abu-Abeid S, Gavert N, Klausner JM, et al. Bariatric surgery in adolescence. J Pediatr Surg 2003;38:1379–1382.
Aggarwal S, Kini SU, Herron DM. Laparoscopic sleeve gastrectomy for morbid obesity: a review. Surg Obes Relat Dis 2007;3:189–194.

Angrisani L, Favretti F, Furbetta F, et al. Obese teenagers treated Lap-Band system: the Italian experience. Surgery 2005;138:877–881.

Ball K, Crawford D, Kenardy J, et al. Longitudinal relationships among overweight, life satisfaction, and aspirations in young women. Obes Res 2004;12:1019–1030.

Barnett SJ, Grimshaw JM, Wells GA, et al. Long-term follow-up and the roll of surgery in adolescents with morbid obesity. Surg Obes Relat Dis 2005;1:394–398.

Chapman AE, Kiroff G, Game P, et al. Laparoscopic adjustable gastric banding in the treatment of obesity: a systematic literature review. Surgery 2004;135:326–351.

Collins J, Mattar S, Qureshi F, et al. Initial outcomes of laparoscopic Roux-en-Y gastric bypass in morbidly obese adolescents. Surg Obes Relat Dis 2007;3:147–152.

Fielding GA, Duncombe JE. Laparoscopic adjustable gastric banding in severely adolescents. Surg Obes Relat Dis 2005;1:399–405.

Freedman DS, Mei Z, Sriniavasan SR, et al. Cardiovascular risk factors and excess adiposity among overweight children and adolescents: the Bogalusa heart study. J Pediatr 2007;150:12–17.

Greenstein RJ, Rabner JG. Is adolescent gastric-restrictive antiobesity surgery warranted? Obes Surg 1995;5:138–144.

Horgan S, Holterman MJ, Jacobsen GR, et al. Laparoscopic adjustable gastric banding for the treatment of adolescent mobid obesity in the United States: a safe alternative to gastric bypass. J Pediatr Surg. 2005;40:86–90.

Kalra M, Inge T, Garcia V, et al. Obstructive sleep apnea in extremely overweight adolescents undergoing bariatric surgery. Obes Res 2005;13:1175–1179.

Lawson ML, Kirk S, Mitchell T, et al. One-year outcomes of Roux-en-Y gastric bypass for morbidly obese adolescents: a multicenter study from the Pediatric Bariatric Study Group. J Pediatr Surg 2006;41:137–143.

Levine MD, Ringham RM, Kalarchian MA, et al. Is family-based behavioral weight control appropriate for severe pediatric obesity? J Eat Disord 2001;30:318–328.

Marcus CL, Curtis S, Koerner CB, et al. Evaluation of pulmonary function and polysomnography in obese children and adolescents. Pediatr Pulmonol 1996;21:176–183.

Mokdad AH, Bowman BA, Ford ES, et al. The continuing epidemics of obesity and diabetes in the United States. JAMA 2002;282:1195–1200.

Nadler EP, Youn HA, Ginsburg HB, et al. Short-term results in 53 US obese pediatric patients treated with laparoscopic adjustable gastric banding. J Pediatr Surg 2007;42:137–141.

Ogden CL, Flegal KM, Carroll MD, et al. Prevalence and trends in overweight among US children and adolescents. JAMA 2002;288:1728–1732.

Papadia FS, Adami GF, Marinari GM, et al. Bariatric surgery in adolescents: a long-term follow-up study. Surg Obes Relat Dis 2007;3:465–468.

Rand CS, Macgregor AM. Adolescents having obesity surgery: a 6-year follow-up. South Med J 1994;87:1208–1213.

Schauer PR, Burguera B, Ikramuddin S, et al. Effect of laparoscopic Roux-en-Y gastric bypass on type 2 diabetes mellitus. Ann Surg 2003;238:467–485.

Silberhumer GR, Miller K, Kriwanek S, et al. Laparoscopic adjustable gastric banding in adolescents: the Austrian experience. Obes Surg 2006;16:1062–1067.

Strauss RS, Bradley LJ, Brolin RE. Gastric bypass surgery in adolescents with morbid obesity. J Pediatr 2001;138:499–504.

Sugerman HJ, Sugerman EL, DeMaria EJ, et al. Bariatric surgery for severely obese adolescents. J Gastrointest Surg 2003;7:102–108.

Yitzhak A, Mizrahi S, Avinoach E. Laparoscopic gastric banding in adolescents. Obes Surg 2006;16:1318–1322.

21. Which Operation Is Best?

Sayeed Ikramuddin
and Gonzalo Torres-Villalobos

A. Introduction

There is no clear consensus as to which is the best operation in bariatric surgery. Perhaps a better question is, "Which is the right operation for the given patient?" No operation is uniformly accepted as the best one. There are too many confounding factors to make this kind of decision making possible. Primarily, the lack of long-term follow-up, established definitions of success, and paucity of randomized data make this unfeasible. In addition, patients may have different goals or biases that determine which operation they choose. Importantly, not all bariatric surgeons perform all bariatric procedures. The preceding sections have reported the outcomes of laparoscopic adjustable banding (LAGB), roux-en-Y gastric bypass (RYGB), sleeve gastrectomy (SG) and the biliopancreatic diversion/duodenal switch (DS) operation. Specific considerations have also been covered for adolescent patients. This chapter attempts to put these data into perspective and offer recommendations that are suitable for a particular patient or clinical circumstance. The appropriate choice of operation begins with a full assessment of the patient's reasons for choosing as well as expectations of weight loss surgery. Information can then be gathered from the history and physical examination, laboratory data, imaging and endoscopic studies, and prior operative notes. Arbitrarily, choice of procedure can be determined by weight, presence of comorbid illness, age, plans of conception, or relevant previous surgery. Collectively, some of these factors can be used to determine a patient's perioperative risk, which might represent an independent way to choose an operation. For example, what would be the best operation for a 26-year-old superobese man with a history of a previous Nissen fundoplication? Certainly even the most singularly aligned surgeon to a particular operation might give pause to the fact that there needs to be particular consideration in this case and that his or her "best" operation, or any operation for that matter, may not be appropriate.

The four most commonly performed procedures for morbid obesity at this time are RYGB, LAGB, DS, and SG. Each procedure has advantages and disadvantages; accordingly, it is important to consider multiple factors when recommending the type of surgery. Few randomized trials exist comparing the different procedures. Algorithms using review of the literature have been developed to match a given patient to a given operation. This algorithm has not yet been tested in a clinical setting and cannot be absolute.

B. Risk

Some patients have severe obesity-related comorbidities that expose them to a high risk of perioperative complications. Many of these patients seek weight loss surgery as they have exhausted medical management. Preoperatively, the strategy for these patients is to reduce this risk. The approach for these high-risk patients includes rigorous goals aiming for weight loss, physical therapy, optimization of medical disorders (diabetes, hypertension, reversible heart disease, etc.) and psychological counseling.

For any high-risk surgical candidate, less extensive, less invasive, and shorter procedures are likely to have lower perioperative morbidity and mortality. Patients with marked comorbidity might be considered for an SG or LAGB because they are technically less complicated and there are no gastrointestinal anastomoses. Morbidly obese individuals with marked comorbidity are considered for sleeve gastrectomy as the first part of a two-stage procedure. Substantial weight loss generated by this restrictive procedure significantly reduces risk associated with the second-stage procedure. A second-stage procedure consisting of an RYGB or DS is performed 6 to 12 months later for long-term weight reduction. The SG has been performed as the sole weight reduction procedure in high-risk patients.

The LAGB can be a good option for patients with marked comorbidities. The procedure is technically simple. Morbidity and mortality are very low, and the length of the procedure is significantly less than other bariatric operations. In addition, LAGB is easier to perform; the absence of an intestinal anastomosis removes the disastrous complication of leak or staple line breakdown in the high-risk morbidly obese patient. A randomized study that compares the outcomes of the SG and LAGB demonstrates that weight loss and loss of feeling of hunger after 1 and 3 years were better after SG than LAGB. GERD was more frequent at 1 year after SG and at 3 years after LAGB. The number of reoperations was important in both groups, but the severity of complications was higher in SG. It is important to remember that there is a finite risk of leakage and bleeding in the SG that far exceeds that seen in the LAGB. Conversely, issues such as slippage do arise long term in this patient population. Outcomes in the sleeve gastrectomy for high-risk patients are limited. In small series outcome was excellent with good resolution of comorbid illness. Studies directly examining the band in patients who are at high risk do not exist.

C. Age

The extremes of age (younger that 18, older than 60 years) remain an area of controversy. With growing awareness of the benefits of bariatric surgery, surgeons are seeing more patients in the extremes of age. The literature dealing with bariatric surgery in the elderly, as in the adolescent population, is sparse. NIH guidelines do not address adolescents.

It is estimated that 25% of US children are obese or overweight, an incidence that has doubled in the last 30 years. In 2004, eligibility criteria for weight loss surgery in this population were suggested (Table 21.1).

Results of both RYGB and LAGB have been retrospectively reviewed in small series of adolescents. The LAGB is attractive because of its low perioperative

Table 21.1. Bariatric surgery for severely overweight adolescents: recommendations.

Presence of severe obesity (BMI >40 kg/m²)
Presence of comorbidities
Skeletal/physiological maturity
Failure of ≥6 months of structured attempts at weight loss
Commitment to evaluation before and after surgery
Commitment and ability to follow nutritional guidelines after surgery
Commitment to avoid pregnancy for ≥1 year postoperatively
Informed consent
Decision-making capacity

Source: Reprinted from Inge TH, Garcia V, Daniels S, et al. A multidisciplinary approach to the adolescent bariatric patient. J Pediatr Surg 2004;39:442–447, with permission from Elsevier.

risk, but long-term data are lacking and there are concerns of the longevity of the device itself. The risk of slippage and erosion appear to increase over time, although changes in the design of the band and refinements in placement techniques may reduce the likelihood of these complications. The RYGB imposes a higher perioperative risk, but it has a longer record of success in weight loss and comorbid resolution. In addition there is some concern in the possibility of long-term metabolic complications. There is a price to pay in terms of iron deficiency and postoperative hypoglycemia (a variant of the dumping syndrome) that must be taken into account. Admittedly it is far easier to manage failed weight loss from a band than that of a gastric bypass. However, some would argue that the band is more likely to fail in this setting. What is clear now is that adolescents should undergo evaluation and treatment at large centers where there is vast experience in bariatric surgery. Adolescents with limited comorbidities may benefit from a multidisciplinary approach incorporating LAGB with behavioral modification techniques. In addition if the LAGB is unsuccessful in these younger patients, later conversion to another procedure can be performed. There is a growing movement to support the use of the SG in this population. Arguments include the elimination of a bypassed stomach and no significant malabsorption; it still remains true that there is a risk of leakage from the staple line that is finite. The claims that this procedure does not have a malabsorptive component still need to be substantiated given the extensive resection of the stomach that is necessary with concomitant removal of intrinsic factor–secreting cell mass. Further, there is still no standardization on how to perform the SG. Many surgeons include the antrum of the stomach in the resection. The antrum plays an important role in reducing the size of food particles. Destruction of the antrum theoretically might lead to increased postoperative nausea. It has been our experience that the follow-up of adolescents is a significant challenge that should not be overlooked. Many factors are responsible for this; younger adolescents need to depend on transportation to be brought in to clinic appointments. Older adolescents struggle because they tend to be highly mobile or attending school, which makes it a struggle to keep appointments.

Likewise, the indication for bariatric surgery for those above age 60 years should be considered on an individual basis. Proof of a favorable risk–benefit ratio must be demonstrated in elderly or ill patients before surgery is contemplated. In elderly patients, the primary objective of surgery is to improve quality of life, even though surgery may be unlikely to increase longevity. Morbidity and mortality for surgery increase with advancing age. In a recent article patients older than 65 years were at a significantly higher risk of death (both early and late) after bariatric surgery. However, it has been demonstrated in many recent studies that both gastric bypass and the LAGB are safe and efficacious in elderly patients. What is clear now is that elder patients should undergo evaluation and treatment at large centers where there is vast experience in bariatric surgery.

Our older patients appear to carry more of a metabolic burden. In this case they would benefit more from RYGB, as it clearly has superior results in terms of remission of type 2 diabetes mellitus (T2DM) and dyslipidemia when cohorts of different studies are compared. For patients with established metabolic disease and who are at very high risk, the role of the SG or LAGB comes into question. In many of these patients anticoagulation must be continued around the time of surgery. This makes procedures such as the SG less attractive. At this time the SG is not covered by Medicare. The LAGB remains an attractive option for these patients.

D. Superobesity

Superobese patients are defined as those with a BMI $\geq 50\,\text{kg/m}^2$. Traditionally complications from bariatric surgery are much higher in this group of patients. The expected average weight loss and weight maintenance increases with the following procedures: LAGB, RYGB, and DS. The mean excess weight losses for these procedures are 48.6%, 68.6%, and 68.8%, respectively. On the contrary, the surgical complexity and potential surgical and long-term metabolic risks of procedures decrease inversely. Subgroup analysis demonstrates that for patients undergoing an RYGB the percent of excess weight loss is lower in heavier patients. The argument remains as to the objective of the surgery—to reduce weight, improve comorbid illness, or both. Admittedly patient satisfaction is a very important consideration. Superobese patients are better candidates for DS or RYGB procedures. The DS is associated with greater weight loss compared with the RYGB and might be a better option for superobese patients. The malabsorptive complications in these patients cannot be ignored. Patients typically have at least three bowel movements per day. The incidence of flatulence and odor is a problem in many of these patients. Also the incidence of revision for malabsorption is 4%. There are few data to support the use of the LABG in the United States for this population.

SG can be done as the first part of a two-stage procedure for long-term weight loss in super-superobese patients, those with a BMI $>60\,\text{kg/m}^2$. Complications associated with laparoscopic DS in super-superobese patients are high. Morbidity has been reported as high as 23% and the mortality as high as 6.5%. Neither open nor laparoscopic one-stage DS has been satisfactory in this group of patients. A second procedure, either RYGB or DS, is performed in the second stage 6 to 12 months after the SG. Important weight loss generated by this restrictive procedure significantly reduces risks associated with the second-stage procedure. It is worrisome that the first-stage operation is susceptible to substantial complications, such as bleeding or leakage.

E. Previous Surgery

1. Nissen fundoplication

Some obese patients present for weight loss surgery having previously undergone antireflux procedures. Several authors have reported their experience with gastric bypass following antireflux procedures and have found that although technically more challenging and carrying a higher risk of morbidity, RYGB is a feasible method for treating obesity and recurrent symptoms of reflux. Some technical considerations must be taken into account, such as the use of pledgets at the first operation, which can make the procedure far more difficult. Some have advocated performing a gastric bypass in these patients by stapling underneath the wrap. Although from a technical point of view this is attractive it results in a grossly enlarged pouch and perhaps a higher theoretical risk of gastric stasis, marginal ulcer, and therefore impaired quality of life in these patients. A modified DS has been proposed, but has compromised weight loss in patients who do not undergo reduction of gastric volume at the same time. A biliopancreatic diversion (BPD) is an option, but this operation has not received acceptance in the United States secondary to the large volume in consumed calories and the multiple number of bowel movements per day. Likely the best course of action for these patients is referral to a center with considerable experience in performing this type of procedure and converting these patients to an RYGB.

2. Colon or small bowel resection

Surgical history can significantly affect surgical morbidity and mortality in a bariatric procedure. Prior abdominal surgery may lead to dense intra-abdominal adhesions that create prohibitive risk for competition of intestinal bariatric procedures. In adhesions, previous intestinal resections, including the ileocecal valve, small bowel, or pylorus, may prevent good evolution of the bariatric procedure or expose the patient to intractable diarrhea or dumping. Accordingly, LAGB may be the safest bariatric procedure in morbidly obese patients with a history of intestinal or colonic resection.

F. Comorbidities

1. Diabetes

T2DM is a common disease associated with morbid obesity. Obesity is the single most important predictor of T2DM. The risk of developing T2DM increases exponentially related to the BMI. Approximately 40% of morbidly obese patients have either impaired fasting glucose or impaired glucose tolerance and nearly 20% have T2DM. Mortality is in the range of 5% per year in morbidly obese diabetics.

The majority of obese patients who undergo bariatric surgery experience a dramatic and usually rapid resolution of T2DM. In the Swedish Obese Subjects study, the largest prospective series reported to date, there was a dramatic decrease in the incidence of T2DM in surgical patients, with 72% at 2 years (odds ratio, 0.14%; 95% confidence interval [CI], 0.08–0.24) and 36% at 10 years (odds ratio, 0.25; 95% CI, 0.17–0.38), confirming that bariatric surgery could prevent new-onset T2DM as well as ameliorate pre-existing disease. The rate of T2DM resolution seemed to vary depending on the type of surgery. Resolution occurs most commonly and rapidly after DS (98%) and RYGB (84%) compared with LAGB (48%). RYGB and DS should be the procedures of choice in patients with T2DM. DS can be considered for higher BMI (superobese patients).

2. Gastroesophageal reflux disease

Gastroesophageal reflux disease (GERD) is extremely common in Western society. Fifteen to twenty percent of adults in the United States experience episodes of GERD. The incidence of GERD in the obese has been reported as high as 72%. A relationship between GERD and increasing BMI has been suggested in females. Some authors have shown a relationship between obesity and estrogen as risk factor for GERD symptoms; there also appears to be an augmentation of this relationship with the addition of postmenopausal hormones. In males, a dose-dependent observation between an increase in BMI and reflux symptoms was observed. Obesity may also increase the severity of GERD. A BMI greater than $35 \, kg/m^2$ is a significant risk factor for developing GERD and esophagitis. Other studies have shown increase in GERD and GERD symptoms in relation to increase in BMI.

There are differences in the outcome of GERD depending on the bariatric procedure. Results of the LAGB are mixed, slippage is known to occur up to 1.5% of the time, and may predispose to GERD. Many studies have shown worsening reflux symptoms after LAGB. Conversely, there are reports of improvement in GERD symptoms after LAGB. RYGB has been deemed to be a beneficial surgical treatment for GERD in the obese population. In theory, a small gastric pouch (15–20 ml) produces little in the way of acid to reflux. By virtue of gastric exclusion, duodenogastroesophageal reflux is rare, making RYGB an ideal operation to correct acid and biliary reflux in the obese population. Fewer data exist for the DS procedure. Certainly bile reflux will be markedly diminished. The effect of DS in GERD remains unclear. Resolution of GERD has been reported after DS.

Despite early resolution of symptoms after LAGB, most patients had a return of reflux symptoms by 6 months, indicating that RYGB may be the procedure of choice for bariatric patients with GERD.

RYGB is a better option in patients with large hiatal hernia and those with paraesophageal hernia or shortened esophagus. Patients with a history of peptic ulcer disease might be better served with LAGB or the DS.

3. Ventral hernia

Many patients who require surgical treatment for morbid obesity also present with abdominal wall hernias. Morbidly obese patients are predisposed to develop ventral hernias, and the risk is even greater than in patients with chronic steroid use. The great majority of ventral hernias are associated with previous abdominal surgeries. Surgeries that require an extensive bowel manipulation, such as RYGB and DS, may need to be done open. For this reason LAGB or SG seem to be attractive options since they do not involve extensive bowel handling.

There is no consensus regarding the optimal treatment of ventral hernias in patients who present for weight loss surgery. Regardless of the prevalence of this challenging clinical problem there is a paucity of literature on this subject. Repair techniques consist of deferred treatment of the ventral hernia until adequate weight loss, or concomitant hernia repair either primarily, or with biodegradable mesh. The issue of simultaneous repair of anterior abdominal wall hernia with mesh during minimally invasive bariatric surgery remains to be answered. Two studies showed that the deferred treatment is dangerous, as it resulted in more than one third of patients developing small bowel obstruction, which required urgent operative management. The reluctance for simultaneous repair is mainly because of the high recurrence rates after primary repair, with a recurrence rate as high as 67%. This is especially true in obese patients. In addition there is contamination related with divided bowel, thus precluding the use of synthetic mesh. Even small hernias (3–4 cm), closed with primarily transfixion transabdominal sutures similar to the technique used for closure of 12-mm trocar sites, are associated with a recurrence rate as high as 22%.

The development of tension-free hernia repair has clearly improved the outcome of ventral hernia repair, by reducing the recurrence rate to a range of 8% to 17% with the use of prosthetic material. Randomized controlled trials have confirmed the superiority of mesh repair over primary repair. The adoption of laparoscopic principles to the Stoppa-Rives method has further improved the treatment of ventral hernias by reducing the recurrence rate to 0% to 3%.

Some articles support the use of biomaterials to concomitant repair of ventral hernias in the patient undergoing laparoscopic RYGB with a very low recurrence rate. The problem of mesh contamination is less for the LAGB because there is no contact with bowel contents. Outcome is less certain.

G. Transplant

Morbid obesity is associated with an increased risk of complications and death in transplant patients. Postoperative weight gain following organ transplantation may in part be explained by a direct corticosteroid effect. Bariatric surgery has been performed after organ transplantation to aid weight loss, improving medical comorbidities, and consequently graft survival. There are a few reports of bariatric surgery in morbidly obese patients, candidates for transplant, and post-transplant patients.

1. Renal transplant

End-stage renal failure is most commonly caused by obesity-related diseases, diabetes mellitus, and essential hypertension, and is best treated with renal transplantation. Also, because operative risks, complications, and death are greater in morbidly obese patients, transplantation may be denied. The major reason for poor outcome in morbidly obese patients after transplantation relates to an increased risk of cardiovascular disease, which is now the leading cause of death in kidney-transplant patients after the first year following transplant. It is well established that diabetes, hypertension, and hyperlipidemia all contribute to the risk of cardiovascular disease and that these complications are exceptionally high both after transplantation and in association with morbid obesity. BMI is a strong independent risk factor for both patient mortality and death-censored graft failure after kidney transplantation.

The potential benefit of RYGB in morbidly obese dialysis and transplant patients has been reported. RYGB leads to a reduction in comorbid conditions that are associated with an increased risk for cardiovascular deaths. In addition RYGB can make previously nontransplantable patients acceptable for transplant. Some series suggest that the indications for RYGB in renal failure and transplant patients should be the same as for the general population.

LAGB can be a good option for patients who are candidates for renal transplant and post-transplant patients. The procedure is technically simple. The morbidity and mortality of the operation are very low, and the length of the procedure is significantly less than other bariatric operations. In addition, LAGB is easier to perform; the absence of intestinal anastomosis removes a disastrous complication from the risk for the high-risk morbidly obese patient. This may be a less attractive option in patients with T2DM.

2. Liver transplant

Obesity is common before and after liver transplantation and has been associated with significant morbidity and mortality. Obesity may cause graft dysfunction through the development of recurrent nonalcoholic steatohepatitis. Liver transplantation has been successfully performed in the morbidly obese. However, wound infection, prolonged ventilatory support, multiorgan failure, and death have been described in the immediate postoperative period. Patients often develop a dramatic increase in weight after liver transplantation.

The feasibility of bariatric surgery in liver transplant recipients is practically unknown. There are some case reports of RYGB in morbidly obese liver transplant recipients with adequate reduction of weight and normalization of liver laboratory tests, lipid profile, diabetes, and hypertension. However, RYGB after liver transplantation can be extremely technically demanding because of adhesions, mostly between the liver and stomach. LAGB in liver transplant patients has not been studied.

H. Other

Patients who crave sweet carbohydrate-rich foods probably benefit from procedures that give a negative biofeedback, such as RYGB. Although superiority of the bypass over the band has not been clearly demonstrated in this population, this is an important consideration. Conversely, for those patients who are compulsive sweet eaters, a minority can develop post–gastric bypass hypoglycemia. Although this can be controlled by diet, it can be a vexing problem to manage.

In patients who need endoscopic surveillance of the stomach, RYGB is contraindicated. The presence of gastric pathology, such as gastric ulcers, polyps, or gastritis with metaplasia, is a relative contraindication for RYGB. The gastric remnant cannot be accessed directly using standard endoscopic techniques in this population. These patients might be better suited for LAGB or DS. This may be an important consideration for those patients who live in areas such as Japan or Chile with increased prevalence of gastric cancer.

Patients who require chronic anti-inflammatory drugs probably benefit from the DS, which is usually nonulcerogenic or LAGB.

Nonalcoholic fatty liver disease occurs in 30% to 100% of obese adults. Nonalcoholic fatty liver disease can lead to cirrhosis and liver failure. Even with this high prevalence, few patients (1.4%) undergoing bariatric surgery have had clinically significant cirrhosis. For any cirrhotic patients undergoing general anesthesia independently of the surgery (except liver transplantation), the overall 30-day mortality has been reported to be as great as 11.6%. In addition, more than 30% of this patient population experienced at least one postoperative complication. The benefits of weight loss surgery must be evaluated considering the potential operative risk in this subset of patients. Surgical weight loss has been associated with both improvement and worsening of liver disease. The malnutrition caused by the rapid weight loss in the early postoperative period can acutely worsen liver function and occasionally might be associated with mortality. Given our lack of understanding and data on the subject and our resultant inability to make informed decisions, it seems prudent to intervene with an operation that would cause the least harm. Shorter and less invasive procedures such as LAGB and SG are likely to result in less risk of worsening liver function in the short and long term. These surgeries are not malabsorptive and have less risk of liver failure compared with the DS. It is unknown how much weight loss is required to achieve optimal improvement in liver function among patients with nonalcoholic fatty liver disease as the etiology of their cirrhosis. Some authors advocate the use of more aggressive procedures such as DS as the first treatment in cirrhotic patients because substantial weight loss after bariatric surgery can lead to considerable improvement in the histologic features of fatty liver disease, reversal of nonalcoholic steatohepatitis, and even true reversal of fibrosis (albeit rare). In many patients the hepatic pathology is related to T2DM. In these patients without synthetic dysfunction the best course of therapy might be to consider RYGB. Of the spectrum of procedures available this has potent resolution of diabetes without the risk of substantial malabsorption. The benefits of bypass for patients with T2DM must be balanced with the risk of variceal bleeding from the gastric remnant, which can be problematic.

I. Conclusion

There are many good operations available to the bariatric surgeon. No operation is universally applicable. A thorough assessment of a patient medical status is paramount in choosing a procedure and should be the basis for operative choice. Those surgeons not performing the "best" match may consider referral to another center.

J. Selected References

Ablassmaier B, Klaua S, Jacobi CA, et al. Laparoscopic gastric banding after heart transplantation. Obes Surg 2002;12(3):412–415.

Abu-Abeid S, Gavert N, Klausner JM, et al. Bariatric surgery in adolescence. J Pediatr Surg 2003;38(9):1379–1382.

Alexander JW, Goodman H. Gastric bypass in chronic renal failure and renal transplant. Nutr Clin Pract 2007;22(1):16–21.

Alexander JW, Goodman HR, Gersin K, et al. Gastric bypass in morbidly obese patients with chronic renal failure and kidney transplant. Transplantation 2004;78(3):469–474.

Almogy G, Crookes PF, Anthone GJ. Longitudinal gastrectomy as a treatment for the high-risk super-obese patient. Obes Surg 2004;14(4):492–497.

Anthony T, Bergen PC, Kim LT, et al. Factors affecting recurrence following incisional herniorrhaphy. World J Surg 2000;24(1):95–100;discussion 1.

Baltasar A, Bou R, Bengochea M, et al. Duodenal switch: an effective therapy for morbid obesity—intermediate results. Obes Surg 2001;11(1):54–58.

Birgisson G, Park AE, Mastrangelo MJ Jr, et al. Obesity and laparoscopic repair of ventral hernias. Surg Endosc 2001;15(12):1419–1422.

Brolin RE, Bradley LJ, Taliwal RV. Unsuspected cirrhosis discovered during elective obesity operations. Arch Surg 1998;133(1):84–88.

Buchwald H. A bariatric surgery algorithm. Obes Surg 2002;12(6):733–746; discussion 47–50.

Buchwald H, Avidor Y, Braunwald E, et al. Bariatric surgery: a systematic review and meta-analysis. JAMA 2004;292(14):1724–1737.

Burger JW, Luijendijk RW, Hop WC, et al. Long-term follow-up of a randomized controlled trial of suture versus mesh repair of incisional hernia. Ann Surg 2004;240(4):578–583; discussion 83–85.

Capella JF, Capella RF. Bariatric surgery in adolescence. is this the best age to operate? Obes Surg 2003;13(6):826–832.

Chu CA GM, Quinn T, et al. Two-stage laparoscopic biliopancreatic diversion with duodenal switch: an alternative approach to super-super morbid obesity. Surg Endosc 2002;16(Abs):S069.

Costanza MJ, Heniford BT, Arca MJ, et al. Laparoscopic repair of recurrent ventral hernias. Am Surg 1998;64(12):1121–1125; discussion 6–7.

Cottam D, Qureshi FG, Mattar SG, et al. Laparoscopic sleeve gastrectomy as an initial weight-loss procedure for high-risk patients with morbid obesity. Surg Endosc 2006;20(6):859–863.

Csendes A, Burgos AM, Smok G, et al. Effect of gastric bypass on Barrett's esophagus and intestinal metaplasia of the cardia in patients with morbid obesity. J Gastrointest Surg 2006;10(2):259–264.

de Jong JR, van Ramshorst B, Timmer R, et al. Effect of laparoscopic gastric banding on esophageal motility. Obes Surg 2006;16(1):52–58.

DeMaria EJ, Sugerman HJ, Kellum JM, et al. Results of 281 consecutive total laparoscopic Roux-en-Y gastric bypasses to treat morbid obesity. Ann Surg 2002;235(5):640–645; discussion 5–7.

Dixon JB, Dixon AF, O'Brien PE. Improvements in insulin sensitivity and beta-cell function (HOMA) with weight loss in the severely obese. Homeostatic model assessment. Diabet Med 2003;20(2):127–134.

Dixon JB, O'Brien PE. Gastroesophageal reflux in obesity: the effect of lap-band placement. Obes Surg 1999;9(6):527–531.

Dolan K, Creighton L, Hopkins G, et al. Laparoscopic gastric banding in morbidly obese adolescents. Obes Surg 2003;13(1):101–104.

Duchini A, Brunson ME. Roux-en-Y gastric bypass for recurrent nonalcoholic steatohepatitis in liver transplant recipients with morbid obesity. Transplantation 2001;72(1):156–159.

Eíd GM, Mattar SG, Hamad G, et al. Repair of ventral hernias in morbidly obese patients undergoing laparoscopic gastric bypass should not be deferred. Surg Endosc 2004;18(2):207–210.

El-Serag HB, Johanson JF. Risk factors for the severity of erosive esophagitis in *Helicobacter pylori*–negative patients with gastroesophageal reflux disease. Scand J Gastroenterol 2002;37(8):899–904.

Fielding GA. Laparoscopic adjustable gastric banding for massive superobesity (>60 body mass index kg/m^2). Surg Endosc 2003;17(10):1541–1545.

Fielding GA, Duncombe JE. Laparoscopic adjustable gastric banding in severely obese adolescents. Surg Obes Relat Dis 2005;1(4):399–405; discussion 7.

Fisher BL, Pennathur A, Mutnick JL, et al. Obesity correlates with gastroesophageal reflux. Dig Dis Sci 1999;44(11):2290–2294.

Flanagan L Jr. Gastric bypass after cardiac transplantation. Obes Surg 1995;5(2):183–185.

Flum DR, Salem L, Elrod JA, et al. Early mortality among Medicare beneficiaries undergoing bariatric surgical procedures. JAMA 2005;294(15):1903–1908.

Forsell P, Hallerback B, Glise H, et al. Complications following Swedish adjustable gastric banding: a long-term follow-up. Obes Surg 1999;9(1):11–16.

Frezza EE, Ikramuddin S, Gourash W, et al. Symptomatic improvement in gastroesophageal reflux disease (GERD) following laparoscopic Roux-en-Y gastric bypass. Surg Endosc 2002;16(7):1027–1031.

Gentileschi P, Kini S, Catarci M, et al. Evidence-based medicine: open and laparoscopic bariatric surgery. Surg Endosc 2002;16(5):736–744.

Gianetta E, Civalleri D, Bonalumi U, et al. [2 cases of death caused by hepatic insufficiency after jejuno-ileal bypass for obesity]. Minerva Chir 1979;34(15–16):1087–1096.

Gomez Escudero O, Herrera Hernandez MF, Valdovinos Diaz MA. [Obesity and gastroesophageal reflux disease]. Rev Invest Clin 2002;54(4):320–327.

Himpens J, Dapri G, Cadiere GB. A prospective randomized study between laparoscopic gastric banding and laparoscopic isolated sleeve gastrectomy: results after 1 and 3 years. Obes Surg 2006;16(11):1450–1456.

Howard RJ, Patton PR, Reed AI, et al. The changing causes of graft loss and death after kidney transplantation. Transplantation 2002;73(12):1923–1928.

Hu FB, Manson JE, Stampfer MJ, et al. Diet, lifestyle, and the risk of type 2 diabetes mellitus in women. NEJM 2001;345(11):790–797.

Inge TH, Garcia V, Daniels S, et al. A multidisciplinary approach to the adolescent bariatric surgical patient. J Pediatr Surg 2004;39(3):442–447; discussion 6–7.

Keeffe EB, Gettys C, Esquivel CO. Liver transplantation in patients with severe obesity. Transplantation 1994;57(2):309–311.

Kellogg TA, Andrade R, Maddaus M, et al. Anatomic findings and outcomes after antireflux procedures in morbidly obese patients undergoing laparoscopic conversion to Roux-en-Y gastric bypass. Surg Obes Relat Dis 2007;3(1):52–57; discussion 8–9.

Kim WW, Gagner M, Kini S, et al. Laparoscopic vs. open biliopancreatic diversion with duodenal switch: a comparative study. J Gastrointest Surg 2003;7(4):552–557.

Lawson ML, Kirk S, Mitchell T, et al. One-year outcomes of Roux-en-Y gastric bypass for morbidly obese adolescents: a multicenter study from the Pediatric Bariatric Study Group. J Pediatr Surg 2006;41(1):137–143; discussion 43.

Leslie D, Kellogg TA, Ikramuddin S. Bariatric surgery primer for the internist: keys to the surgical consultation. Med Clin North Am 2007;91(3):353–381, x.

Liakakos T, Karanikas I, Panagiotidis H, et al. Use of Marlex mesh in the repair of recurrent incisional hernia. Br J Surg 1994;81(2):248–249.

Locke GR 3rd, Talley NJ, Fett SL, et al. Risk factors associated with symptoms of gastroesophageal reflux. Am J Med 1999;106(6):642–649.

Luyckx FH, Desaive C, Thiry A, et al. Liver abnormalities in severely obese subjects: effect of drastic weight loss after gastroplasty. Int J Obes Relat Metab Disord 1998; 22(3):222–226.

Mattar SG, Velcu LM, Rabinovitz M, et al. Surgically-induced weight loss significantly improves nonalcoholic fatty liver disease and the metabolic syndrome. Ann Surg 2005;242(4):610–617; discussion 8–20.

Meier1 Kriesche HU, Arndorfer JA, Kaplan B. The impact of body mass index on renal transplant outcomes: a significant independent risk factor for graft failure and patient death. Transplantation 2002;73(1):70–74.

Mognol P, Chosidow D, Marmuse JP. Laparoscopic sleeve gastrectomy as an initial bariatric operation for high-risk patients: initial results in 10 patients. Obes Surg 2005;15(7): 1030–1033.

Nair S, Verma S, Thuluvath PJ. Obesity and its effect on survival in patients undergoing orthotopic liver transplantation in the United States. Hepatology 2002;35(1):105–109.

Nilsson M, Johnsen R, Ye W, et al. Obesity and estrogen as risk factors for gastroesophageal reflux symptoms. JAMA 2003;290(1):66–72.

Patterson EJ, Davis DG, Khajanchee Y, et al. Comparison of objective outcomes following laparoscopic Nissen fundoplication versus laparoscopic gastric bypass in the morbidly obese with heartburn. Surg Endosc 2003;17(10):1561–1565.

Pontiroli AE, Folli F, Paganelli M, et al. Laparoscopic gastric banding prevents type 2 diabetes and arterial hypertension and induces their remission in morbid obesity: a 4-year case-controlled study. Diabetes Care 2005;28(11):2703–2709.

Pories WJ, Swanson MS, MacDonald KG, et al. Who would have thought it? An operation proves to be the most effective therapy for adult-onset diabetes mellitus. Ann Surg 1995;222(3):339–350; discussion 50–52.

Prachand VN, Davee RT, Alverdy JC. Duodenal switch provides superior weight loss in the super-obese (BMI > or =50 kg/m^2) compared with gastric bypass. Ann Surg 2006;244(4):611–619.

Raftopoulos I, Awais O, Courcoulas AP, et al. Laparoscopic gastric bypass after antireflux surgery for the treatment of gastroesophageal reflux in morbidly obese patients: initial experience. Obes Surg 2004;14(10):1373–1380.

Regan JP, Inabnet WB, Gagner M, et al. Early experience with two-stage laparoscopic Roux-en-Y gastric bypass as an alternative in the super-super obese patient. Obes Surg 2003;13(6):861–864.

Reich D, Rothstein K, Manzarbeitia C, et al. Common medical diseases after liver transplantation. Semin Gastrointest Dis 1998;9(3):110–125.

Rios A, Rodriguez JM, Munitiz V, et al. Factors that affect recurrence after incisional herniorrhaphy with prosthetic material. Eur J Surg 2001;167(11):855–859.

Sarr MG. Is a bariatric procedure appropriate in patients with portal hypertension secondary to cirrhosis? Surg Obes Relat Dis 2006;2(3):405–406, discussion 6–7.

Schauer PR, Burguera B, Ikramuddin S, et al. Effect of laparoscopic Roux-en-Y gastric bypass on type 2 diabetes mellitus. Ann Surg 2003;238(4):467–484; discussion 84–85.

Schauer PR, Ikramuddin S. Laparoscopic surgery for morbid obesity. Surg Clin North Am 2001;81(5):1145–1179.

Schuster R, Curet MJ, Alami RS, et al. Concurrent gastric bypass and repair of anterior abdominal wall hernias. Obes Surg 2006;16(9):1205–1208.

Sjostrom L, Lindroos AK, Peltonen M, et al. Lifestyle, diabetes, and cardiovascular risk factors 10 years after bariatric surgery. NEJM 2004;351(26):2683–2693.

Spivak H, Hewitt MF, Onn A, et al. Weight loss and improvement of obesity-related illness in 500 U.S. patients following laparoscopic adjustable gastric banding procedure. Am J Surg 2005;189(1):27–32.

Strauss RS, Bradley LJ, Brolin RE. Gastric bypass surgery in adolescents with morbid obesity. J Pediatr 2001;138(4):499–504.

Strignano P, Collard JM, Michel JM, et al. Duodenal switch operation for pathologic transpyloric duodenogastric reflux. Ann Surg 2007;245(2):247–253.

Sugerman HJ, DeMaria EJ, Kellum JM, et al. Effects of bariatric surgery in older patients. Ann Surg 2004;240(2):243–247.

Sugerman HJ, Kellum JM Jr, Reines HD, et al. Greater risk of incisional hernia with morbidly obese than steroid-dependent patients and low recurrence with prefascial polypropylene mesh. Am J Surg 1996;171(1):80–84.

Suter M, Dorta G, Giusti V, et al. Gastric banding interferes with esophageal motility and gastroesophageal reflux. Arch Surg 2005;140(7):639–643.

Tichansky DS, Madan AK. Laparoscopic Roux-en-Y gastric bypass is safe and feasible after orthotopic liver transplantation. Obes Surg 2005;15(10):1481–1486.

Varela JE, Wilson SE, Nguyen NT. Outcomes of bariatric surgery in the elderly. Am Surg 2006;72(10):865–869.

Wang Y. Cross-national comparison of childhood obesity: the epidemic and the relationship between obesity and socioeconomic status. Int J Epidemiol 2001;30(5):1129–1136.

Weiss H, Nehoda H, Labeck B, et al. Organ transplantation and obesity: evaluation, risks and benefits of therapeutic strategies. Obes Surg 2000;10(5):465–469.

Willett WC, Dietz WH, Colditz GA. Guidelines for healthy weight. NEJM 1999;341(6): 427–434.

Wilson LJ, Ma W, Hirschowitz BI. Association of obesity with hiatal hernia and esophagitis. Am J Gastroenterol 1999;94(10):2840–2844.

Zimmet P, Alberti KG, Shaw J. Global and societal implications of the diabetes epidemic. Nature 2001;414(6865):782–787.

Ziser A, Plevak DJ, Wiesner RH, et al. Morbidity and mortality in cirrhotic patients undergoing anesthesia and surgery. Anesthesiology 1999;90(1):42–53.

IV. Complications

22. Anastomotic Leaks after Laparoscopic Gastric Bypass

Alexander Perez and Eric J. DeMaria

A. Background

Anastomotic leak is a rare early complication of laparoscopic gastric bypass surgery and is an independent risk factor for mortality.[1]

B. Incidence

Leak rates range from 0% to 5.2% in contemporary series (Table 22.1).

1. Factors associated with increased risk of anastomotic leak

Older, heavier male patients with multiple comorbid conditions, limited surgical experience, open approach, antecolic approach, stapled closure, single-layer closure, and revisional surgery.

2. Factors associated with a decreased risk of anastomotic leak

Increased surgical experience, laparoscopic approach, retrocolic approach, hand-sewn closure, double-layer closure, use of reinforcing the anastomosis with peristrip sor fibrin sealant, and use of Robot-assisted approach.

C. Diagnosis

Intraoperative endoscopic pneumatic testing facilitates early identification of leaks.

The majority of patients will present within the first 3 days after surgery with tachycardia, fever, and/or abdominal pain. These nonspecific symptoms may be delayed or more subtle compared with nonobese patients. Laboratory findings are also nonspecific and usually consist of leukocytosis.

Persistent tachycardia and tachypnea may occur before a temperature elevation or impressive leukocytosis and the differential may include pulmonary

Table 22.1. Incidence of leaks after laparoscopic gastric bypass.[a]

Author	Institution	Year	n	Incidence
DeMaria EJ	Virginia Commonwealth University	2002	281	4.6%
Fernandez AZ Jr	Virginia Commonwealth University	2004	554	4.2%
Csendes A	University Hospital Santiago Chile	2005	557	2.1%
Schweitzer MA	Johns Hopkins Medical Institute	2006	251	0%
Sekhar N	Vanderbilt University	2006	340	0%
Kligman M	University of Maryland	2007	257	0.8%
Edwards MA	Medical College of Georgia	2007	353	4.8%
Lee S	Virginia Commonwealth University	2007	1,080	5.2%
Gonzalez R	Multi-institution[b]	2007	1,539	2.1%
Nguyen NT	University Health-System Consortium[c]	2007	1,6357	1.4%

[a] Series with more than 100 patients to avoid learning curve effect.
[b] University of South Florida Health Sciences Center, Mayo Clinic, Rochester, Emory University, Cleveland Clinic Florida.
[c] UHC is an alliance of 97 academic medical centers and 153 of their affiliated hospitals, representing 90% of the nation's nonprofit academic medical centers.

embolism. The patient's weight limits the diagnostic modalities available. Many institutions use an upper GI series (UGI) in search of extravasation of contrast and subsequently computed tomography (CT) to determine feasibility of draining a fluid collection or after an inconclusive UGI study in the face of symptoms suggestive of an anastomotic leak. Use of UGI and CT to detect leaks has been well documented in this setting. UGI found leaks 30%, CT found leaks 56%, and combined found leaks 70% of the time in one published report. When a leak is identified it is mostly from a single source and predominantly at the gastrojejunostomy, and less likely from the remnant stomach or jejunojejunostomy. These leaks may be contained or drain freely into the left upper abdominal quadrant. Initial UGI did not detect 9/10 jejunojejunostomy leaks in one series and the median detection time was longer in the jejunojejunostomy leak group than the gastrojejunostomy leak group. Patients with normal studies may harbor leaks, especially at the jejunojejunostomy or excluded stomach. Normal study findings should not delay therapy if clinical signs suggest a leak.

D. Management

Many patients with leaks may be managed successfully nonoperatively with nothing by mouth, antibiotics, CT-guided drainage, and TPN.

Others may require surgery with either open or laparoscopic repair of leak, anastomotic revision or resection, drainage, and placement of a gastrostomy tube in the remnant stomach for postoperative nutrition.

Several of these of patients require intubation for respiratory insufficiency and transfer to the ICU to manage multisystem organ failure.

E. Outcome

Long-term morbidity and mortality associated with leaks include wound infection, gastrogastric fistula, and death (6% to 22%). The average length of stay is 18 to 28 days.

At 18 months after surgery percent excess body weight loss was 71%. Mortality rate from gastrojejunostomy leaks was 2.3%. Jejunojejunostomy leak was associated with a 40% mortality rate.

F. Conclusion

Anastomotic leaks after laparoscopic gastric bypass are rare but potentially lethal. Meticulous attention to surgical technique including a linear-stapled, double-layered hand-sewn gastrojejunostomy with oversewing of the gastric remnant, intraoperative endoscopic insufflation, and methodical postoperative approach to search for leaks with routine UGI with selective CT and high clinical suspicion, will reduce the incidence of leaks and the associated morbidity and mortality.

G. Selected References

Blachar A, Federle MP, Pealer KM, et al. Gastrointestinal complications of laparoscopic Roux-en-Y gastric bypass surgery: clinical and imaging findings. Radiology 2002;223(3):625–632.

Buckwalter JA, Herbst CA. Complications of gastric bypass for morbid obesity. Am J Surg 1980;139(1):55–60.

Carucci LR, Turner MA, Conklin RC, et al. Roux-en-Y gastric bypass surgery for morbid obesity: evaluation of postoperative extraluminal leaks with upper gastrointestinal series. Radiology 2006;238(1):119–127.

Csendes A, Burdiles P, Burgos AM, et al. Conservative management of anastomotic leaks after 557 open gastric bypasses. Obes Surg 2005;15(9):1252–1256.

DeMaria EJ, Sugerman HJ, Kellum JM, et al. Results of 281 consecutive total laparoscopic Roux-en-Y gastric bypasses to treat morbid obesity. Ann Surg 2002;235:640–647.

Edwards MA, Jones DB, Ellsmere J, et al. Anastomotic leak following antecolic versus retrocolic laparoscopic Roux-en-Y gastric bypass for morbid obesity. Obes Surg 2007;7(3):292–297.

Fernandez AZ, DeMaria EJ, Tichansky DS, et al. Experience with over 3,000 open and laparoscopic bariatric procedures: multivariate analysis of factors related to leak and resultant mortality. Surg Endosc 2004;18(2):193–197.

Fernandez AZ, DeMaria EJ, Tichansky DS, et al. Multivariate analysis of risk factors for death following gastric bypass for treatment of morbid obesity. Ann Surg 2004;239(5):698–703.

Gonzalez R, Haines K, Gallagher SF, et al. Does experience preclude leaks in laparoscopic gastric bypass? Surg Endosc 2006;20(11):1687–1692.

Gonzalez R, Sarr MG, Smith CD, et al. Diagnosis and contemporary management of anastomotic leaks after gastric bypass for obesity. J Am Coll Surg 2007;204(1):47–55.

Gorecki P, Wise L, Brolin RE, et al. Complications of combined gastric restrictive and malabsorptive procedures: Part 1. Curr Surg 2003;60(2):138–144.

Jamal MK, DeMaria EJ, Johnson JM, et al. Impact of major co-morbidities on mortality and complications after gastric bypass. Surg Obes Relat Dis 2005;1(6):511–516.

Kligman MD. Intraoperative endoscopic pneumatic testing for gastrojejunal anastomotic integrity during laparoscopic Roux-en-Y gastric bypass. Surg Endosc 2007;21(8):1403–1405.

Lee S, Carmody B, Wolfe L, et al. Effect of location and speed of diagnosis on anastomotic leak outcomes in 3828 gastric bypass cases. J Gastrointest Surg 2007;11(6):708–713.

Madan AK, Lanier B, Tichansky DS. Laparoscopic repair of gastrointestinal leaks after laparoscopic gastric bypass. Am Surg 2006;72(7):586–591.

Marshall JS, Srivastava A, Gupta SK, et al. Roux-en-Y gastric bypass leak complications. Arch Surg 2003;138(5):520–524.

Mason EE, Printen KJ, Hartford CE, et al. Optimizing results of gastric bypass. Ann Surg 1975;182(4):405–414.

Matthews BD, Sing RF, DeLegge MH, et al. Initial results with a stapled gastrojejunostomy for the laparoscopic isolated roux-en-Y gastric bypass. Am J Surg 2000;179(6):476–481.

Nguyen NT, Hinojosa M, Fayad C, et al. Use and outcomes of laparoscopic versus open gastric bypass at academic medical centers. J Am Coll Surg 2007;205(2):248–255.

Schweitzer MA, Lidor A, Magnuson TH. A zero leak rate in 251 consecutive laparoscopic gastric bypass operations using a two-layer gastrojejunostomy technique. J Laparoendosc Adv Surg Tech A 2006;16(2):83–87.

See C, Carter PL, Elliott D, Mullenix P, Eggebroten W, Porter C, Watts D. An institutional experience with laparoscopic gastric bypass complications seen in the first year compared with open gastric bypass complications during the same period. Am J Surg 2002;183(5):533–538.

Sekhar N, Torquati A, Lutfi R, et al. Endoscopic evaluation of the gastrojejunostomy in laparoscopic gastric bypass. A series of 340 patients without postoperative leak. Surg Endosc 2006;20(2):199–201.

Shauer P, Ikramuddin S, Hamad G, et al. The learning curve for laparoscopic Roux-en-Y gastric bypass is 100 cases. Surg Endosc 2003;17:212–215.

Silecchia G, Boru CE, Mouiel J, et al. Clinical evaluation of fibrin glue in the prevention of anastomotic leak and internal hernia after laparoscopic gastric bypass: preliminary results of a prospective, randomized multicenter trial. Obes Surg 2006;16(2):125–131.

Yu J, Turner MA, Cho SR, et al. Normal anatomy and complications after gastric bypass surgery: helical CT findings. Radiology 2004;231(3):753–760.

Yu SC, Clapp BL, Lee MJ, et al. Robotic assistance provides excellent outcomes during the learning curve for laparoscopic Roux-en-Y gastric bypass: results from 100 robotic-assisted gastric bypasses. Am J Surg 2006;192(6):746–749.

23. Gastric Bypass: Gastrointestinal Bleeding

Ross L. McMahon

A. Introduction

Gastrointestinal bleeding can be a complication of any gastrointestinal surgery. However, in bariatric surgery, and Roux-en-Y gastric bypass surgery in particular, gastrointestinal bleeding can cause symptoms in the postoperative period that are similar to other common postoperative complications (pulmonary embolism, leak/sepsis). The incidence of postoperative GIH after laparoscopic GBP ranges from 0.8% to 9.4%. In a recent series of 155 patients who underwent laparoscopic Roux-en-Y gastric bypass, the incidence of GIH was 3.2%.

Prompt recognition of bleeding, as well as prompt identification of site, allows the bariatric surgeon to tailor the management of the patient and avoid unnecessary tests and procedures.

B. Etiology

Postoperative gastrointestinal bleeding after Roux-en-Y gastric bypass can be categorized by the time frames in which it occurs as acute, subacute, or chronic. Acute bleeding generally occurs within 72 hours of surgery. Subacute bleeding can occur beyond 72 hours, but should occur within 30 days of surgery. Chronic bleeding generally occurs after 30 days.

Classification of postoperative bleeding according to the time frame of its presentation is helpful because it points to the possible etiology of the hemorrhage. It should be noted that cases of bleeding in the chronic postoperative phase (beyond 30 days) may also be "acute" in the sense that serious, life-threatening hemorrhage may occur. Again, the classification scheme of acute, subacute, and chronic is useful primarily in assessment of possible diagnoses and treatment strategies for postoperative GI bleeding. The patient's condition, including hemodynamics and serial blood counts, should guide assessment of the severity and "acuteness" of the hemorrhage itself.

1. Acute bleeding

Bleeding within the first 72 hours after surgery is usually the result of bleeding from the staple lines or suture lines; vessels within the cut tissue are not compressed adequately by staple lines or suture to overcome the blood pressure within them. In the Roux-en-Y gastric bypass, there are three prime locations for staple line/suture line bleeding: the gastric pouch-jejunostomy site, jejunostomy site, and excluded stomach.

Conditions that make a staple line leak more likely include: anticoagulation medications (warfarin, heparin, low-molecular-weight heparin), antiplatelet medications (aspirin, nonsteroidal anti-inflammatory drugs [NSAIDs], clopidogrel), the thickness of the tissue, staple leg length, and tissue gap.

Other less common causes of acute gastrointestinal bleeding after Roux-en-Y gastric bypass are the following:

- Acute or chronic (previously undetected) gastric or duodenal ulcer in either the gastric pouch or excluded stomach
- Gastritis
- Undetected submucosal tumor necrosis

2. Subacute bleeding

Bleeding occurring 72 hours to 30 days is less often caused by failure of staple/suture line hemostasis, and more commonly from a gastric or duodenal ulcer. Other sources may be gastritis, NSAID gastropathy, bleeding secondary to anticoagulation, and, less commonly, erosion of a band in the case of banded Roux-en-Y gastric bypass.

3. Chronic bleeding

Bleeding occurring beyond 30 days encompasses causes of subacute bleeding and adds other causes. Like subacute bleeding, chronic gastrointestinal bleeding (GIB) can be the result of gastric or duodenal bleeding. However, Roux-en-Y gastric bypass–specific causes of GIB must also be entertained; this includes marginal ulcer (usually on the jejunal side of the gastrojejunostomy) and gastrogastric fistula. Other sources may be erosion of a band in the case of banded Roux-en-Y gastric bypass, gastritis, and NSAID gastropathy. Other causes of gastrointestinal bleeding, unrelated to the Roux-en-Y gastric bypass, must also be considered when occurring distantly from the primary operation.

Iron deficiency anemia is a risk after Roux-en-Y gastric bypass, as malabsorption of ingested iron in the diet occurs. Hematocrit should be followed at least on an annual basis for the rest of the patient's life. Iron deficiency may develop from chronic GI blood loss due to blood lost from menstruation in women. Serious anemia may not be correctable with oral iron supplementation due to malabsorption issues, and parenteral iron may be required. Hormonal therapy to reduce/eliminate menses or even hysterectomy is occasionally necessary. Postoperative iron supplementation is recommended for menstruating women after gastric bypass. Blood donation may also be inadvisable.

C. Diagnosis

1. Acute bleeding

In general, the cardinal signs of bleeding in the early postoperative period are the same in morbidly obese patients as they are in any surgical patient. Specifically, the symptoms most commonly associated with bleeding are tachycardia, hypotension, and low urine output. These can be easily confused with a leak or pulmonary embolism; however, a CBC usually points quite clearly in the direction of bleeding when it is present. The source site of the bleeding can be an area of ambiguity.

Traditional diagnostic modalities, such as endoscopic evaluation, should be used this early after surgery only if absolutely necessary and with great care to avoid causing visceral distention, anastomotic disruption, and subsequent suture line leakage. In addition to the effects of the blood loss itself, major intraluminal bleeding early after RYGB can lead to a transient obstruction from clotting at the distal (jejunojejunal) anastomosis. This, in turn, can lead to proximal intraluminal distension and increased risk of perforation of the gastric remnant or at the proximal (gastrojejunal) anastomosis.

2. Subacute bleeding

Upper GI bleeding after the first postoperative week is most commonly associated with erosion or ulceration from excessive restriction or band erosion after banded Roux-en-Y gastric bypass, and from anastomotic ulceration after Roux-en-Y gastric bypass. It is also commonly associated with gastritis, erosion, or ulceration from NSAIDs. Evaluation is primarily by upper GI endoscopy. In Roux-en-Y gastric bypass, patients in whom no bleeding site is seen on upper endoscopy, it may be useful to repeat the procedure with a long endoscope/colonoscope to examine the jejunojejunal anastomosis and common channel. Due to the anatomy of the Roux-en-Y, it is often difficult to visualize the gastric remnant, but the indirect evidence of blood at the distal anastomosis or in the common channel selectively would implicate a distal gastric or duodenal source.

D. Treatment

Treatment of gastrointestinal bleeding in the acute setting depends on the nature and severity of the GI bleed. The stability of the patient's hemodynamic status is the key determinant in whether to intervene or not. Hemodynamic instability includes blood pressure drop, despite adequate resuscitation, and global or regional perfusion that is not adequate to support normal organ function.

Fortunately, in many circumstances, nonoperative treatment is possible and appropriate. Nonoperative therapy of bleeding includes fluid resuscitation, frequent vitals, monitoring urine output, and stopping or even reversing anticoagulation. Frequent reassessment of the patient's hemodynamic status should be performed. Indications for operative treatment include failure of nonoperative treatment, ongoing transfusion requirements, or instability.

Treatment of gastrointestinal bleeding caused by ulcers, gastritis, or erosions after Roux-en-Y gastric bypass is similar to that in nonoperated patients, with endoscopic intervention as needed, cessation of NSAID use, PPI therapy, and identification and eradication, if associated with *H. pylori* infection. At the time of upper endoscopy, it is particularly useful to look for evidence of bile reflux into the gastric pouch or proximal Roux limb. In the presence of bile reflux, there may be a yellow tint of the intraluminal fluid. It may also be useful to collect fluid from the gastric pouch for pH measurement. If the pH of the gastric fluid is less than 3, treatment with additional PPI dosing is indicated. If the gastric pouch pH is at least 4, however, additional PPIs are less likely to have therapeutic benefit and treatment with sucralfate suspension (1 g two to four times daily, as tolerated) in combination with any established PPI regimen may be more likely to be successful. Note that Sucralfate should not be taken within an hour of a PPI, iron, or calcium supplementation, so it is occasionally difficult for these patients to tolerate a QID schedule for this drug. Given the risk of recurrent bleeding, follow-up endoscopy in 8 to 12 weeks to assess healing and hemostasis at the bleeding source is indicated to guide further therapy.

Chronic gastrointestinal bleeding after Roux-en-Y gastric bypass often occurs as a result of the same pathological processes that cause acute bleeding, albeit in a milder form. The evaluation should proceed in a similar fashion, starting with upper endoscopy. However, because obesity is associated with an increased risk of colorectal cancer, in the absence of an identifiable upper source of blood loss, evaluation of occult blood loss or isolated iron deficiency should include colonoscopy.

E. Prevention

The prevention of gastrointestinal bleeding can be grouped into technical and nontechnical strategies. Nontechnical strategies include ensuring adequate time off ASA, Plavix, or other platelet-inhibiting drugs. Ensuring adequate INR off warfarin will also reduce the risk of gastrointestinal bleeding in patients on that drug. Postoperative patients on warfarin will have limited oral intake of vitamin K in their diet; therefore, the dose of warfarin will have to be reduced and the INR carefully monitored. This should be done weekly or even biweekly in the postoperative period to avoid over anticoagulation. Depending on the indication, consideration should be given to if and when to reintroduce warfarin. If it is feasible to be off it for a period of time postoperatively, this should reduce the risk of gastrointestinal bleeding. Obviously, this can only be done when the indications for warfarin allow a delay in reintroduction.

Technical strategies to reduce gastrointestinal bleeding include: oversewing staple lines, use of smaller staple leg lengths, generous use of clipping, intraoperative endoscopy, and the use of staple line reinforcement sleeves.

Traditional gastrointestinal surgery concepts suggest that small bowel anastomoses should be performed using 3.5-mm staple leg lengths (blue load). Bariatric surgeons modified this approach to using 2.5-mm (white) staple leg lengths to reduce bleeding. Similarly, gastric stapling was traditionally undertaken with 4.8-mm (green) cartridge. Most Bariatric surgeons today use 3.5-mm (blue) loads for stapled transaction in creating the proximal gastric pouch. Today's variety in available staples allows customization of the staple leg length to reduce the size of the formed staple to improve tissue compression and, ultimately, hemostasis.

Intraoperative endoscopy is often used to check for leaks at the gastrojejunostomy. A convenient side benefit of endoscopy is that it allows one to visualize the gastric pouch intraluminal staple line and gastrojejunostomy anastomosis. Sometimes, significant bleeding can be identified and located, allowing intraoperative correction with suture over sew techniques.

Staple line reinforcement buttressing materials are a recent adjunct device that might reduce the chances of a leak at the staple line. Many have made the observation that bleeding at the external staple line appears to be less common with these materials, requiring fewer clip applications. This has led investigators to hypothesize that staple line reinforcement may lead to a reduced incidence of gastrointestinal bleeding. Unfortunately, since the incidence of postoperative gastrointestinal bleeding is relatively low, the number of patients required to be recruited into a study to determine a reduction in gastrointestinal bleeding is very large. To date, no sufficiently powered study has been published showing definitive evidence that staple line reinforcement materials reduce gastrointestinal bleeding. Studies have shown a reduction in intraoperative bleeding and a reduced requirement for clip application and oversewing. One study showed an 84% reduction in staple line bleeding sites at gastric tissue, an 83% reduction in staple line bleeding sites at jejunal tissue, and a 100% reduction in staple line bleeding sites at mesenteric tissue with the use of the staple line reinforcement sleeves.

F. Conclusion

Gastrointestinal bleeding is a potentially life-threatening complication of Roux-en-Y gastric bypass. It has an incidence after Roux-en-Y gastric bypass of approximately 3%. Fortunately, most of these cases can be treated nonoperatively. However, knowledge of the likely causes enables the bariatric surgeon to attack the problem in a structured fashion, minimizing the risk to the patient. Prevention strategies, including staple line reinforcement, although in the early stages of assessment, show promise.

G. Selected References

Abell TL, Minocha A. Gastrointestinal complications of bariatric surgery: diagnosis and therapy. Am J Med Sci 2006;331(4):214–218.

Consten EC, Gagner M, Pomp A, et al. Decreased bleeding after laparoscopic sleeve gastrectomy with or without duodenal switch for morbid obesity using a stapled buttressed absorbable polymer membrane. Obes Surg 2004;14(10):1360–1366.

Kaplan LM. Gastrointestinal management of the bariatric surgery patient. Gastroenterol Clin North Am 2005;34(1):105–125.

Nguyen NT, Longoria M, Welbourne S, et al. Glycolide copolymer staple–line reinforcement reduces staple site bleeding during laparoscopic gastric bypass: a prospective randomized trial. Arch Surg 2005;140(8):773–778.

Papasavas PK, Caushaj PF, McCormick JT, et al. Laparoscopic management of complications following laparoscopic Roux-en-Y gastric bypass for morbid obesity. Surg Endoscop 2003;17:610–614.

Shahriari A, Hinder RA, Stark ME, et al. Recurrent severe gastrointestinal bleeding complicating treatment of morbid obesity. J Clin Gastroenterol 2000;31(1):19–22.

24. Intestinal Obstruction after Laparoscopic Gastric Bypass

Alexander Perez and Eric J. DeMaria

A. Background

Intestinal obstruction is a rare complication of laparoscopic gastric bypass surgery, which if not identified and managed promptly, may result in gangrenous bowel, sepsis, and subsequent death.

B. Incidence

Intestinal obstruction rates range from 1.5% to 5.2% in contemporary series (Table 24.1).

C. Etiology of Intestinal Obstruction

The majority of intestinal obstruction after laparoscopic gastric bypass is secondary to internal hernias, adhesions, and kinking of the jejunojejunostomy (Table 24.2).

D. Diagnosis

The clinical presentation of intestinal obstruction after laparoscopic gastric bypass typically includes abdominal pain (82–86%), nausea (49%), vomiting (47–67%), and occasionally all three combined (28%). A small quantity of clear emesis or dry heaving is more likely because of the small gastric pouch. When bilious emesis is present, obstruction at or distal to the jejunojejunostomy should be suspected.

Laboratory findings such as leukocytosis (23%) are rare and nonspecific. Time to presentation varies greatly from 1 day to several years postoperatively. Seventy percent of patients in one series presented within the first postoperative year.

Radiologic work-up includes plain abdominal films (35% positive for obstruction), UGI (33–55% positive for obstruction), and CT (48–90% positive for obstruction). A mesenteric swirl on CT is a reliable indicator of internal hernia after laparoscopic Roux-en-Y gastric bypass (sensitivity 61–83% and specificity 67–94%).

Table 24.1. Incidence of intestinal obstruction after laparoscopic Roux-en-Y gastric bypass.

Author	Institution	Year	n	Incidence
DeMaria EJ	Virginia Commonwealth University	2002	281	1.5%
Felsher J	Cleveland Clinic Foundation	2003	115	5.2%
Champion JK	Videoscopic Institute of Atlanta	2003	711	1.8%
Nguyen NT	University of California, Irvine	2004	225	4%
Hwang RF	Advanced Bariatric Center, Fresno, CA	2004	1,715	3%
Carmody B	Virginia Commonwealth University	2005	785	2.5%
Cho M	Cleveland Clinic Florida	2006	1,400	1.5%
Husain S	University of Rochester	2007	2,325	4.4%
Escalon A	Pontificia Universidad Catolica de Chile	2007	754	4.7%

Table 24.2. Etiology of intestinal obstruction after laparoscopic gastric bypass.

Etiology	Percent of total
Internal hernia	12–54%
Adhesions	14–38%
Roux limb stricture at mesocolic window	8–21%
Kinking at jejunojejunostomy	4–29%
Kinking at gastrojejunostomy	4%
Port-site hernia	2–4%
Obstruction at jejunojejunostomy	1–2%
Narrowing at jejunojejunostomy	7%
External compression at transverse colon	1–4%
Incarcerated ventral hernia	1–24%
Intussusception	5%

E. Sequential Intraoperative Prevention of Intestinal Obstruction

While the open approach to gastric bypass has been associated with less likelihood of obstruction secondary to internal hernias, the laparoscopic approach provides less incidence of intestinal obstruction secondary to adhesions.

An antecolic Roux limb position reduces the incidence of intestinal obstruction by avoiding internal hernias at the colonic mesentery (0.4–1.8% vs. 3.7–9.3%). In the setting of an excessively foreshortened jejunal mesentery, a retrocolic Roux limb position with closure of the mesocolic defect should be performed with nonabsorbable sutures. Care must be taken to avoid excessive narrowing of the Roux limb through the transverse mesocolon.

The jejunal mesentery should be divided down to its base in order to lengthen the Roux limb mesentery to avoid tension on the gastrojejunostomy and subsequent external compression of the transverse mesocolon in an antecolic approach.

The jejunojejunostomy is created with the firing of a 60-mm–long cartridge with a 2.5-mm staple height for a wide patent anastomosis and improved hemostasis, thus avoiding obstruction by intraluminal blood clot. A hand-sewn closure or stapled closure should be done by avoiding narrowing the anastomosis by incorporating excessive tissue. Close the jejunal mesenteric defect to avoid an internal hernia at the jejunojejunostomy and employ an "antiobstruction stitch" to prevent kinking at this site.

Regardless of antecolic or retrocolic Roux limb position Peterson's space should be closed. A double layer gastrojejunostomy with an outer hand-sewn running layer will help prevent kinking at the gastrojejunostomy.

Close all port sites larger than 10 mm or use radial dilating ports. Repair a ventral hernia with suture or bioabsorbable mesh during gastric bypass to avoid subsequent intestinal obstruction.

F. Management

Due to a vague clinical presentation, nonspecific laboratory abnormalities, and potentially negative radiologic work-up, a low threshold must be to explore patients with clinically suspicious presentations and those who fail to improve clinically.

Laparoscopic exploration is feasible in nearly all patients after laparoscopic gastric bypass (83–100%) with intraoperative bypass of the site of obstruction, reduction of internal hernia, lysis of adhesions, or gastric bypass revision. Low conversion rates have been reported (7–17%), and bowel resection is required very rarely if exploration is performed promptly (2–8%).

G. Outcome

There have been recurrences (4.8–18%) after laparoscopic management of intestinal obstruction after gastric bypass. Mortality rates associated with intestinal obstruction are fortunately low (0–8%), indicative of successful early intervention.

H. Conclusion

Intestinal obstruction after laparoscopic gastric bypass is a rare but potentially lethal complication of laparoscopic gastric bypass. This may present anytime, from immediately after surgery to many years postoperatively. Meticulous attention to surgical technique with an antecolic approach when possible and closure of all mesenteric defects, ventral hernias, and port sites larger than 10 mm, along with a methodical postoperative approach to evaluation of intestinal obstruction facilitated by high clinical suspicion, UGI, and CT, will reduce the associated morbidity and mortality.

I. Selected References

Brolin RE. The antiobstruction stitch in stapled Roux-en-Y enteroenterostomy. Am J Surg 1995;169(3):355–357.

Capella RF, Iannace VA, Capella JF. Bowel obstruction after open and laparoscopic gastric bypass surgery for morbid obesity.
J Am Coll Surg 2006;203(3):328–335.

Carmody B, DeMaria EJ, Jamal M, et al. Internal hernia after laparoscopic Roux-en-Y gastric bypass. Surg Obes Relat Dis 2005;1(6):543–548.

Champion JK, Williams M. Small bowel obstruction and internal hernias after laparoscopic Roux-en-Y gastric bypass. Obes Surg 2003;13(4):596–600.

Cho M, Carrodeguas L, Pinto D, et al. Diagnosis and management of partial small bowel obstruction after laparoscopic antecolic antegastric Roux-en-Y gastric bypass for morbid obesity. J Am Coll Surg 2006;202(2):262–268.

DeMaria EJ, Sugerman HJ, Kellum JM, et al. Results of 281 consecutive total laparoscopic Roux-en-Y gastric bypasses to treat morbid obesity. Ann Surg 2002;235(5):640–645.

Eid GM, Collins J. Application of a trocar wound closure system designed for laparoscopic procedures in morbidly obese patients. Obes Surg 2005;15(6):871–873.

Eid GM, Mattar SG, Hamad G, et al. Repair of ventral hernias in morbidly obese patients undergoing laparoscopic gastric bypass should not be deferred. Surg Endosc 2004;18(2):207–210.

Escalona A, Devaud N, Pérez G, et al. Antecolic versus retrocolic alimentary limb in laparoscopic Roux-en-Y gastric bypass: a comparative study. Surg Obes Relat Dis 2007;3(4):423–427.

Felsher J, Brodsky J, Brody F. Small bowel obstruction after laparoscopic Roux-en-Y gastric bypass. Surgery 2003;134(3):501–505.

Higa KD, Ho T, Boone KB. Internal hernias after laparoscopic Roux-en-Y gastric bypass: incidence, treatment and prevention. Obes Surg 2003;13(3):350–354.

Husain S, Ahmed AR, Johnson J, et al. Small-bowel obstruction after laparoscopic roux-en-y gastric bypass: etiology, diagnosis, and management. Arch Surg 2007;142(10):988–993.

Hwang RF, Swartz DE, Felix EL. Causes of small bowel obstruction after laparoscopic gastric bypass. Surg Endosc 2004;18(11):1631–1635.

Iannelli A, Facchiano E, Gugenheim J. Internal hernia after laparoscopic Roux-en-Y gastric bypass for morbid obesity. Obes Surg 2006;16(10):1265–1271.

Johnson WH, Fecher AM, McMahon RL, et al. VersaStep trocar hernia rate in unclosed fascial defects in bariatric patients. Surg Endosc 2006;20(10):1584–1586.

Lockhart ME, Tessler FN, Canon CL, et al. Internal hernia after gastric bypass: sensitivity and specificity of seven CT signs with surgical correlation and controls. AJR Am J Roentgenol 2007;188(3):745–750.

Nelson LG, Gonzalez R, Haines K, et al. Spectrum and treatment of small bowel obstruction after Roux-en-Y gastric bypass. Surg Obes Relat Dis 2006;2(3):377–383.

Nguyen NT, Huerta S, Gelfand D, et al. Bowel obstruction after laparoscopic Roux-en-Y gastric bypass. Obes Surg 2004;14(2):190–196.

Rogula T, Yenumula PR, Schauer PR. A complication of Roux-en-Y gastric bypass: intestinal obstruction. Surg Endosc 2007 Sept 22 [Epub ahead of print].

Schweitzer MA, DeMaria EJ, Broderick TJ, et al. Laparoscopic closure of mesenteric defects after Roux-en-Y gastric bypass. J Laparoendosc Adv Surg Tech A 2000;10(3):173–175.

25. Roux-en-Y Gastric Bypass: Stomal Stenosis

Janey S.A. Pratt

A. Introduction

Stomal stenosis is simply an anastomotic stricture at the gastrojejunal anastomosis of a Roux-en-Y gastric bypass (RYGB). It is one of the common postoperative complications of RYGB. The incidence is reported between 3.1% and 15.7%, depending on the type of anastomosis used. The method of anastomosis seems to have the greatest impact on the formation of stomal stenosis. It appears that the greatest risk of stenosis is conferred by use of a 21-mm circular stapler, followed in order by a 25-mm circular stapler, linear stapler, and handsewn anastomosis. There have been several studies showing no difference in weight loss between the different anastomotic methods. At least one major study shows no relationship between stomal stenosis and antecolic versus retrocolic anastomoses. There also is no gender, comorbidity, or BMI relationship to stomal stenosis. Stomal stenosis is significantly more common after revisional surgery.

The cause of stomal stenosis has not been scientifically proved; however, most believe that it is related to excessive scar formation or ischemia. Another possible cause is recurrent vomiting; however, since vomiting is one of the symptoms of stenosis, it is impossible to determine which came first. Finally, stomal stenosis can be associated with gastric/marginal ulcers, anasamotic banding, or with "pursestringing" of permanent suture material. In the case on concurrent ulcer disease stomal stenosis occurs late and may be caused by smoking or NSAID use.

Presenting symptoms include dysphagia, solid food intolerance, nausea, and vomiting. Presentation is usually 1 to 2 months postoperatively. Late presentation (>4 months) suggests concurrent pathology, such as ulcer, band material, or retained suture material.

B. Diagnosis

The diagnosis of a stricture can usually be made by taking a careful history, however sometimes it is confused by the patient who is learning to eat slowly. Patients describe tolerating most liquids but vomiting with solids. They describe pain behind the sternum after eating that is only relieved by vomiting. If they are cutting their food small and eating slowly and still have these symptoms then further intervention is warranted. A Barium swallow may be helpful, especially if a 1-cm barium tablet is used, but it is only diagnostic, whereas EGD can be both diagnostic and allow for concurrent therapeutic intervention. Most surgeons make the diagnosis by EGD, which allows for identification of suture material or ulcer, that can be removed or treated (respectively) prior to endoscopic dilatation.

C. Treatment

Dilatation of stomal stenosis is the treatment of choice and is successful after one time in 55% to 83% of cases. Repeat dilations are indicated if symptoms persist or recur, and until it is felt that there is no progress being made, in which case surgery is indicated. Most endoscopists prefer an esophageal balloon dilator or an anastomotic balloon dilator, passed via flexible endoscopy. Dilatation to a size of 15 to 20 mm is standard, but 18 mm is the most common size used. Savary-Gilliard dilators can also be used; some feel they are more effective. Postdilation microperforations are uncommon and usually can be treated conservatively. Surgical revision for stomal stenosis is indicated in cases of complete obstruction, band errosion or recidivism, despite endoscopic dilatation.

Strictures in the setting of prior Banding or banded RYGB should be treated differently. Often, an experienced endoscopist can tell at endoscopy if the band or the anastamosis is the site of the stricture. Dilatation of a stricture at the banding site is controversial due to the risk of erosion of the band. If a Marlex or Prolene mesh was used, it is unlikely to respond to dilation, and surgery should be considered early. If there is a silastic ring or an adjustable band, then dilatation risks exposing the band and should be used with caution or to treat simple edema. If the band is already exposed, then revision, including removal of the band, is indicated. Removal of an eroded band via endoscopic cutting techniques may be possible in some patients.

D. Selected References

Ahmad J, Martin J, Ikramuddin S, et al. Endoscopic balloon dilation of gastroenteric anastomotic stricture after laparoscopic gastric bypass. Endoscopy 2003;35:725–728.

Escalona A, Devaud N, Boza C, et al. Gastrojejunal anastomotic stricture after Roux-en-Y gastric bypass: ambulatory management with the Savary-Gilliard dilator. Surg Endosc 2007;21:765–768.

Giotein D, Papasavas PK, Gagne D, et al. Gastrojejunal strictures following laparoscopic Roux-en-Y gastric bypass for morbid obesity. Surg Endosc 2005;19:628–632.

Nguyen NT, Stevens CM, Wolfe BM. Incidence and outcome of anastomotic stricture after laparoscopic gastric bypass. J Gastrointest Surg 2003;7(8):997–1003.

Takata MC, Ciovica R, et al. Predictors, treatment and outcomes of gastrojejunostomy stricture after gastric bypass for morbid obesity. Obes Surg 2007;17(7):878–884.

26. Gastric Bypass: Marginal Ulceration

Bradley J. Needleman

A. Introduction

Since its introduction, the ulcerogenic potential of the Roux-en-Y gastric bypass has been brought into question. Despite concerns stemming from the high incidence of stomal ulceration in previous gastric exclusion operations, this has not been found to be the case with Roux-en-Y gastric bypass, which excludes much of the acid-secreting mucosa, as well as the antrum. Mason et al. postulated that gastric acid secretion is under antral control in most people; therefore, gastric bypass operations decrease acid production. This was further demonstrated by Smith et al., who documented significantly decreased basal and pentagastrin-stimulated acid production in the gastric pouch.

Despite the predicted reduction in acid secretion, marginal ulceration can be a relatively troublesome complication of Roux-en-Y gastric bypass, with a historical incidence reported to be between 3% and 20%, and more recent literature reporting an incidence between 2% and 4%.

B. Etiology

Marginal ulcerations usually occur on the jejunal side of the gastrojejunal anastomosis and may be the result of jejunal exposure to acid. Jejunal mucosa does not possess the protective mechanisms normally found in the duodenum, normally the first part of the small intestine exposed to acid. The etiology of marginal ulcers in the bariatric population is complex and may involve a combination of factors that include an increase in acid production, the breakdown of mucosal defenses, and technical nuances of the operation. Factors that have been suggested or shown to influence the formation of marginal ulcers include:

1. Nonsteroidal anti-inflammatory medications (NSAIDs)
2. Tobacco
3. Ischemia
4. *H. pylori*
5. Alcohol
6. Foreign body reaction (nonabsorbable suture or staples)
7. Large or vertically oriented pouch
8. Gastrogastric fistula
9. Predominant vagal stimulation of gastric acid secretion

C. Clinical Presentation and Diagnosis

The diagnosis and treatment of marginal ulceration must include a careful history and physical examination, including the signs and symptoms distinguishing it from other clinical manifestations and complications common after gastric bypass, and identifying conditions requiring urgent intervention. Marginal ulcers may present at any time from months to years after the initial operation, and patients will typically complain of pain, nausea, dysphagia, and in contrast to peptic ulcer disease, pain aggravated by eating. In addition, patients may present with symptoms of chronic or acute GI bleeding and perforation that may require emergent intervention. Interestingly, these symptoms do not seem to correlate well to the size and depth or number of ulcers found.

The diagnosis of a marginal ulcer may be made on the basis of clinical presentation and treated empirically or confirmed with endoscopic and/or radiographic studies. Upper endoscopy is considered the best diagnostic tool in making the diagnosis and characterizing marginal ulcers. Upper GI contrast studies may also be useful, especially in aiding in the diagnosis of gastrogastric fistula, large gastric pouch, and outlet obstruction. Differential diagnoses in these patients include stricture, internal hernia, biliary colic, bowel obstruction, pancreatitis, and non-compliance with dietary guidelines.

It is important to identify and limit factors that cause and may prevent healing of ulcers, including NSAIDs, alcohol, and tobacco use. Testing for *H. pylori* is appropriate and treatment advisable if positive. If marginal ulcer persists despite optimal medical management, further diagnostic testing may be necessary to rule out ulcerogenic anatomic issues, including gastrogastric fistulas, large or horizontally oriented gastric pouch that might contain large amounts of parietal cells, and the presence of foreign bodies in the ulcer base, such as nonabsorbable sutures or staples.

D. Medical Treatment

Once the diagnosis of marginal ulceration is made, treatment includes acid suppression, as well as treatment of the underlying cause, if it is identified. Removal of agents known to be ulcerogenic, eradication of *H. pylori*, if present, and treatment with proton pump inhibitors and sucralfate often promptly improve the patient's symptoms and promote resolution of the ulcer. Duration of treatment is not clearly defined, but some studies suggest 6 to 12 months or longer after resolution of symptoms. Repeat upper endoscopy may be helpful to evaluate and document success or failure of treatment.

E. Surgical Treatment

Surgical intervention for marginal ulceration after gastric bypass may be necessary in patients who have acute complications or are symptomatic and/or refractory to optimal medical management. Indications for emergent operative intervention include active bleeding and acute perforation. Symptomatic patients, who have failed optimal medical management, being considered for surgical intervention need a complete work-up to rule out causative factors (i.e., smoking, NSAIDs, *H. pylori*, prednisone), presence of foreign material in the ulcer base, gastrogastric fistula, or excessive pouch size. A tailored surgical approach may be required, depending on the results of this evaluation. Several surgical options are described for the treatment of marginal ulcer and its complications.

1. Resection and revision of gastrojejunostomy

    a. Revision of the gastrojejunostomy may be necessary in the patient who has ongoing and debilitating symptoms from nonhealing ulcers (pain, dysphagia, nausea, and stricture). Revision of the gastrojejunostomy in this setting includes:

- Open or laparoscopic approach that includes resection of the gastrojejunostomy to include the small bowel segment containing the ulcer, partial gastric resection to resize the pouch, if excessively large, and recreating the gastrojejunostomy via the surgeon's preferred method.
- May be combined with vagotomy
- May be combined with a gastrostomy tube placement in distal gastric remnant

2. Vagotomy

    a. A subset of patients that do not respond as expected to the acid-reducing nature of the gastric bypass may have abnormal vagal innervation of the pouch, as described by Mason et al. In this subset of patients, vagotomy with or without excision of the distal stomach has been found to be an effective treatment of nonhealing or recurrent ulceration.

Options may include:

- Truncal or highly selective vagotomy via abdominal approach
- Truncal vagotomy via right thoracoscopy

3. Treatment of acute perforation

    a. Surgical options should be guided by a number of factors, including: size of perforation, amount of contamination, clinical condition of patient, and etiology of the perforation.

Options for treatment include:

- Open or laparoscopically placed omental patch and/or oversew of perforation
- Resection of the gastrojejunostomy to include the small bowel segment containing the ulcer, gastric resection to reduce the pouch size, if excessively large, and re-creating the gastrojejunostomy via the surgeon's preferred method

- May be combined with vagotomy
- Consideration for placing a gastrostomy tube in distal gastric remnant

4. Closure of gastrogastric fistula

a. Gastrogastric fistulas (staple line disruptions) allow secretions from the remnant stomach to reflux into the gastric pouch and increase the jejunum's exposure to acid, causing erosion and ulceration. Marginal ulcer due to gastrogastric fistula is often refractory to medical treatment and the fistula may contribute to weight regain. Symptomatic gastrogastric fistulas may require intervention. Several options for treatment include:

- Flexible endoscopic approach to closing the fistula with endoluminal suture/clips and/or the injection of fibrin sealant tissue adhesives. Temporary endoscopic stenting may prove to be an adjunct to this approach.
- Open or laparoscopic approach with identification of the fistula tract between the pouch and distal stomach. Separation of the pouch from distal remnant via resection of the fistulous tract by stapling or over-sewing. Placement of omentum or Roux limb interposition between the pouch and distal stomach.
- Resection of the distal gastric remnant.
- May be combined with vagotomy.

5. Endoscopic removal of foreign bodies

a. When suture material or metal staples are found in the base of a persistent marginal ulcer, it may be prudent to attempt endoscopic removal. Several techniques have been described to endoscopically cut and remove these foreign bodies from the ulcer base.

F. Conclusions

Marginal ulceration can be a particularly morbid complication after Roux-en-Y gastric bypass. Although the etiology in many patients is not clear, technical considerations, postoperative behaviors, and prophylaxis may all be helpful in reducing the incidence of marginal ulceration. In the operating room, creating a small pouch, dividing the stomach, optimizing Roux limb perfusion, and avoiding nonabsorbable materials when possible seem prudent when performing Roux-en-Y gastric bypass. Counseling patients to avoid potentially ulcerogenic agents after surgery, including NSAIDs, tobacco, and excesses of alcohol, should be standard for any weight loss surgery program. In addition, prophylaxis of patients with a proton pump inhibitor for 2 months to a year or longer after initial operation may be beneficial in prevention of marginal ulceration and their complications. There is some evidence to suggest a role for preoperative endoscopy in all bariatric surgery patients undergoing gastric bypass.

G. Selected References

Capella JF, Capella RF. Staple disruption and marginal ulceration in gastric bypass procedures for weight loss. Obes Surg 1996;6:44–49.

Dallal RM, Bailey LA. Ulcer disease after gastric bypass. Surg Obes Relat Dis 2006;2: 455–459.

Gumbs AA, Duffy AJ, Bell RL. Incidence and management of marginal ulceration after laparoscopic Roux-en-Y gastric bypass. Surg Obes Relat Dis 2006;2:460–463.

Mason EE, Munns JR, Kealey GP, et al. Effect of gastric bypass on gastric secretion. Am J Surg 1977;131:162–168.

Pope GD, Goodney PP, Burchard KW, et al. Peptic ulcer/stricture after gastric bypass: a comparison of technique and acid suppression variables. Obes Surg 2002;12:30–33.

Sacks BC, Mattar SG, Qureshi FG, et al. Incidence of marginal ulcers and the se of absorbale anastomotic sutures in laparoscopic Roux-en-Y gastric bypass. Surg Obes Relat Dis 2006;2:11–16.

Schirmer B, Erenoglu C, Miller A. Flexible endoscopy in the management of patients undergoing Roux-en-Y gastric bypass. Obes Surg 2002;12:634–638.

Smith CD, Herkes SB, Behrns KE, et al. Gastric acid secretion and Vitamin B12 absorption after vertical Roux-en-Y gastric bypass for morbid obesity. Ann Surg 1993;1:91–96.

Wilson JA, Romagnuolo J, Byrne KT, et al. Predictors of endoscopic findings after Roux-en-Y gastric bypass Am J Gastroenterol 2006;101:2194–2199.

27. Laparoscopic Adjustable Gastric Banding: Infection, Slippage, and Hiatal Hernia

Marina Kurian

A. Introduction

Laparoscopic adjustable banding surgery has increased due to popularity with patients and bariatric surgeons. Long-term management of these patients should include careful questioning of the patients for troublesome symptoms, a low threshold for further testing, and careful physical examination. Infection of the gastric band or the reservoir port usually presents early after band placement. Gastric prolapse or "band slippage" can occur early or late. Hiatal hernia usually presents later in the postoperative period after the band has been adjusted.

B. General Guidelines for Postoperative Follow-up

1. Schedule of office visits

Patients are usually seen monthly for the first year, every 2 to 3 months for the second year, and then 6 months to yearly thereafter. Obviously, if there is an issue, the patient should be seen sooner than their scheduled visit.

2. Routine radiologic imaging

A baseline study after gastric banding is helpful, as it allows comparison with subsequent delayed imaging studies. A limited barium upper GI series is often obtained prior to the first adjustment to delineate the postgastric banding anatomy.

3. Worrisome signs and symptoms

    a.   Skin discoloration at the port site. Immediately after the surgery, the port site can be bruised and the incision slightly red. If the port site incision appears increasingly red or dark or becomes increasingly indurated or tender, cellulitis or deeper soft tissue infection may be present.

Drainage from the wound is unusual, and should be carefully evaluated as a sign of possible infection.

b. Fevers or recurrent low-grade temperatures. Early or late in the postoperative period, fevers may be evaluated with a CBC with differential. CXR and CT scan of the abdomen may reveal abnormalities (including pleural effusion) if a band infection or abscess is suspected. Gastric band erosion can also cause low-grade temperature or fever, but is best evaluated by upper endoscopy.

c. Persistent vomiting. The patient should be questioned regarding how rapidly they eat, how long they chew food before swallowing, and even the amount of "stress" they are experiencing in their day-to-day lives. Patients may vomit more frequently when they are not making appropriate food choices and/or eating rapidly, and this is indicative of a possible behavioral explanation, rather than a band-related complication. The band can feel more "tight" to the patient during periods of stress, resulting in more frequent vomiting. If none of the above applies, or if symptoms persist despite counseling, the patient should have a reduction in fill volume.

d. Inability to tolerate liquids or saliva. This is an emergency that requires removal of fluid and a limited contrast upper GI series to assess the esophagus, stomach, and band position. This level of symptomatic high-grade obstruction occasionally occurs without a change in the band position or abnormality of the esophagus/stomach or contrast X-ray evaluation. If there is no abnormality, these patients can be gradually re-adjusted. If gastric prolapse is identified or suspected, surgical management may be necessary.

e. Persistent heartburn. Heartburn in the band patient is not usually related to acid reflux but to food stasis within the stomach and esophagus above the band. Occasional heartburn may occur when food transiently obstructs the band lumen, and is not usually of concern. More frequent heartburn and heartburns that occur when the patient is not eating, or with every meal should prompt removal of some fluid from the band. Heartburn that occur when patients lie down immediately after eating may be relieved by withholding food and liquid 2 hours before bedtime. Occasionally, postnasal drip can generate heartburn when there is no ingestion of food, and this should respond to treatment with a decongestant. If after removal of some fluid from the band the patient still has heartburn, an esophagram should be ordered.

f. Persistent reflux or nocturnal reflux. After banding, patients may reflux ingested food or drink. Reflux can occur normally after overeating, but the patient is usually cognizant of having taken in too much. If the reflux occurs with very small amounts of food, the patient likely needs some fluid out of the band. Nocturnal reflux can manifest in several different ways, including night cough. The patient may complain of burning in the chest or throat, a bitter taste in the mouth, or fluid coming out of the nose and mouth that awakens her or him from sleep. Nocturnal reflux requires removal of some fluid from the band. If symptoms do not resolve, an esophagram should be obtained.

4. Diagnostic radiologic imaging

a. Compare the band axis to the baseline study. A band that becomes more horizontal or changes its axis 90 degrees or more may be indicative of a gastric prolapse.

b. Evaluate using contrast ingestion for the presence of a hiatal hernia.

c. Compare the amount of stomach above the band to the baseline UGI contrast study. If there is significant overhang of the stomach around the band profile, a gastric prolapse is likely. Sometimes, there can be concentric or asymmetric pouch dilation (different entities from a prolapse), and overhang of the stomach around the band is usually not present in the former conditions.

d. Evaluate for esophageal dysmotility or dilation.

5. Upper endoscopy

a. May need to remove fluid from the band and/or be prepared to use a pediatric endoscope (usually not needed).

b. Performed with caution if a gastric prolapse is suspected. May be done to be sure the stomach and prolapsed portion of the stomach are decompressed.

c. Need to retroflex to document erosion. Look for visible suture and/or visible band, often yellow- or green-tinted color.

d. Appropriate and safe to perform if trying to diagnose a gastric ulcer, gastritis, or bleeding ulcer.

C. Port Infection

The port can become infected early or late. Not every port infection is a band (intra-abdominal component) infection. Early infection may manifest as redness over the port site. The redness may, in fact, be due to a port hematoma or a seroma at the site. An early infection should be treated with antibiotics for 1 to 2 weeks. If there is a draining seroma, the site should be cleaned twice a day with an antibacterial cleanser (i.e., Betadine, Hibiclens) and kept dry. The patient should be started on an antibiotic for skin flora prophylactically. An antibacterial ointment (Bacitracin, Neosporin) can be applied also, depending on the surgeon's preference. If there is a palpable seroma, it can be aspirated. The patient should be seen weekly for evaluation until the redness or drainage is resolved.

If infection recurs after the antibiotic course is completed, the port should be removed and cultured. To accomplish this, I prefer to make a separate incision cephalad to the port, and just above where the tubing enters the abdominal wall. I prefer to culture the tubing in this location, away from the port site incision. The tubing can be clipped or tied off and then cut with the abdominal portion dropped into the peritoneal cavity. Next I close this incision and then open the port site incision to remove and culture the port. Alternatively, laproscopy can be performed, and the tubing can be cut and cultured followed by removal of the port. The antibiotic course should be tailored to the organism that grows, and the patient should be treated for a further 2 weeks. If the culture is negative, I treat the patient for a total of 7 to 10 days. If the culture of the tubing grows organisms, there is a strong chance that the band is infected, and a discussion should be undertaken with the patient to discuss removal of the intra-abdominal component, although some surgeons would manage the patient expectantly.

A late port site infection should also be treated with antibiotics to see if it clears. The surrounding area should be examined for any scratches, rashes, or pustules, which might suggest a possible etiology of the infection. If no obvious skin lesion is present, the patient should be questioned regarding low-grade fevers and be scheduled for an upper endoscopy specifically looking for erosion. The endoscopy should be performed by a gastroenterologist or surgeon who is familiar with the device and with findings of band erosion. If there is no evidence of erosion and the infection clears with antibiotics, the patient can be managed expectantly. However, if the infection recurs, the port will need to be removed and the site cultured as described. Again, the antibiotics should be tailored to the organism(s) identified, and a full course of treatment instituted.

After approximately 2 to 3 months, the port can be replaced at a different site, and the tubing of the band should be recultured. Some surgeons would re-site the port at the time of initial port removal. To do so, I would recommend dividing the tubing intra-abdominally (e.g., via laparoscopy), culturing the tubing, and then re-site the port prior to removing the infected port via open incision.

D. Band Infection

The intra-abdominal component of the gastric band can develop an early or late infection. In the early postoperative period, patients may present with peritonitis and fevers. Patients may also present with port infections that fail to clear despite antibiotics. The gastric band should be removed, cultured, and the stomach and esophagus tested for leak either with methylene blue or with an air leak test via intraoperative endoscopy. Antibiotics appropriately adjusted based on cultures should be administered for at least 2 weeks.

A late band infection may also present as a port infection, intra-abdominal abscess, peritonitis, or gastric erosion. The band should be removed, cultured, and even if there is no known erosion, the stomach should be tested as described to rule out leak. Occasionally, a late band infection is related to an indolent staphylococcal infection, and the band will have to be removed. In early or late band infection, once the band is removed, the band can generally be replaced in about 3 months.

E. Gastric Prolapse or "Band Slippage"

Gastric prolapse occurs in up to 5% of patients after adjustable gastric banding and refers to the prolapse (or herniation) of gastric fundus in a cephalad direction through the band. Prolapse can be an anterior prolapse of the anterior/lateral part of the fundus or a posterior prolapse of the posterior part of the fundus. Anterior prolapse is most common with the pars flaccida technique and partial gastrogastric suturing.

Patients present with inability to swallow liquids and sometimes their own saliva. They can also have persistent vomiting or nighttime reflux. Some patients also regurgitate undigested food. These scenarios arise from gastric outlet obstruction. Patients may also present with left chest or upper abdominal pain, and this may be an indication for urgent surgery since the prolapsed portion of the stomach can become ischemic and necrotic. Sometimes, the patient's condition can be improved by removing the fluid from the band. The patient with persistent pain and inability to tolerate secretions requires emergent operation. In the majority of cases, the band can be repositioned after all the adhesions are divided and the prolapse reduced. Some surgeons just cut the band out and reposition a new band higher. Most of these cases (>98%) may be completed laparoscopically.

At the time of revision, some surgeons perform a gastric plication of the fundus below the level of the band to increase the bulk of the fundus and prevent it from prolapsing through the band during the primary operation. This has decreased the incidence of gastric prolapse through the band but has not completely prevented it. After reduction of prolapse, it is important to test the stomach for a leak with either an air leak test via an endoscope or by methylene blue. Once revision is completed, it is also important to check the integrity of the band system by accessing the port and instilling saline to see if there is a leak of fluid in the system.

F. Hiatal Hernia

Surgeons are advised to look for a hiatal hernia at the time of gastric banding surgery. A hiatal hernia may be identified preoperatively on an imaging study. A moderate to large hiatal hernia is visualized as soon as the left lobe of the liver is raised. A hiatal hernia is suspected intraoperatively if a dimple or defect at the anterior esophageal hiatus is visualized. A hiatal hernia may be identified during the posterior dissection of the right crus. If a widening of the hiatus is identified posteriorly, it is important to ascertain if some of the retroperitoneal fat at the hiatus is extending into the mediastinum. If there is a fat pad extending into the mediastinum, it must be reduced to ensure that there is no sliding component of hiatal herniation. The peritoneal attachments should be divided. If there is a moderate to large hiatal hernia, the gastrohepatic ligament should be divided and the peritoneal sac reduced or divided circumferentially followed by completion of the crural repair.

A hiatal hernia may develop in a patient following gastric banding. Symptoms include heartburn and/or reflux worsening with progressive tightening of the band. Symptoms may resolve when the band is loosened. Postoperative hiatal hernia is problematic when there is inadequate weight loss with less fluid in the band or if symptoms do not resolve with removal of fluid from the band. Such patients require revision of the band with reduction and repair of the hiatal hernia and repositioning of the band. Full mobilization of the esophagus after division of the gastrohepatic ligament, division or reduction of the peritoneal sac, takedown of the gastrogastric suturing and repositioning of the band are necessary components of the revision procedure. At least 2 to 3 cm of intra-abdominal esophagus should be present at completion of the procedure. A leak test should be performed following the procedure for both the areas of dissection (stomach and esophagus) and the port system itself.

Crural repair can be performed anteriorly or posteriorly, or both. Generally, if there is a moderate to large hiatal hernia, the crural repair is performed posteriorly.

G. Pouch Dilation

Gastric pouch dilation after gastric banding is usually concentric, but infrequently can be asymmetric. The symptoms of pouch dilation are similar to hiatal hernia and gastric prolapse to some degree. Patients complain of frequent heartburn and reflux and require fluid to be removed from the band. An esophagram (obtained because of persistent symptoms despite fluid removal or recurrent symptoms with attempts at readjustment) shows a large pouch or an increased volume of stomach above the band compared with previous studies. If the band axis has not changed and there is no "overhang" of stomach over the band profile, the diagnosis is usually pouch dilation. Asymmetric pouch dilation is a less frequent finding, but also characterized by no change in the band axis, yet only part of the pouch is dilated. Pouch dilation should be treated with a trial of band deflation and a liquid diet for 2 to 4 weeks. Then an esophagram should be obtained, although some surgeons might slowly reinflate the band. Recurrent symptoms, inadequate weight loss, or recurrent heartburn/reflux suggest the band position should be reversed surgically. Operative findings typically show circumferential pouch dilation without gastric prolapse. A hiatal hernia may be present and should be identified and fixed during the revision. Pouch dilation can recur again despite the repositioning and patients should be made aware of this before selecting band revision over conversion to another bariatric operation (e.g., gastric bypass). In general, symptoms improve after the band is repositioned.

H. Postoperative Imaging

After an intra-abdominal procedure to reposition the band, band replacement, or hiatal hernia repair, a new baseline limited upper GI series should be obtained to document band and stomach anatomy. Confirming the absence of leak is an added benefit, although a negative esophagram should not outweigh clinical suspicions if a leak is suspected by the patient's course. In this setting, re-exploration is superior to contrast examination.

I. Selected References

Boschi S, Fogli L, Berta RD, et al. Avoiding complications after laparoscopic esophago-gastric banding: experience with 400 consecutive patients. Obes Surg 2006;16(9):1166–1170.

Favretti F, Segato G, Ashton D, et al. Laparoscopic adjustable gastric banding in 1,791 consecutive obese patients: 12 year results. Obes Surg 2007;17(2):168–175.

Lyass S, Cunneen SA, Hagiike M, et al. Device-related reoperations after laparoscopic adjustable gastric banding. Am Surg 2005;71(9):738–743.

Moser F, Gorodner MV, Galvani CA, et al. Pouch enlargement and band slippage: two different entities. Surg Endosc 2006;20(7):1021–1029.

Parikh MS, Laker S, Weiner M, et al. Objective comparison of complications resulting from laparoscopic bariatric procedures. J Am Coll Surg 2006;202(2):252–261.

Ponce J, Fromm R, Paynter S. Outcomes after laparoscopic adjustable gastric band repositioning for slippage or pouch dilation. Surg Obes Relat Dis 2006;2(6):627–631.

28. Gastric Erosion Following Adjustable Gastric Banding

Helmuth T. Billy

A. Gastric Erosion

Laparoscopic placement of an adjustable gastric band has proven to be one of the safest surgical procedures for the surgical treatment of obesity. Adjustable gastric banding is a relatively simple, short surgical procedure with a low complication rate. Additional advantages include adjustability of the stoma, as well as easy reversibility and preservation of the inherent anatomy of the GI tract. The disadvantage of adjustable gastric banding includes the presence of a foreign body with an inherently higher susceptibility to infections complications. Gastric erosion is a significant and severe complication associated with adjustable gastric banding.

Penetration of the gastric wall following Lap Band placement can occur both acutely, within a few weeks of operation; or late, as it can be seen months or years following successful implantation of the device. Once a diagnosis of erosion has been made, the definitive surgical treatment is removal of the device.

B. Incidence and Etiology

Rates of erosion following adjustable gastric banding have ranged from 0% to 14%. Most series report erosion rates between 0.5% and 1% (Table 28.1). The occurrence of gastric erosion is a rare complication and falls into two categories of presentation, early and late. Early erosions occur within weeks to 6 months of implantation. Late band erosion presents more than 6 months following implantation and can be discovered years following what appeared to be a successful gastric banding operation.

Early erosions are generally considered to occur following undetected gastric trauma during operative dissection and placement of the band. Undetected gastric or esophageal perforation or injury can present with early peritonitis and require emergent operative intervention. Meticulous and careful surgical dissection with judicious use of electrocautery may avoid surgical trauma as a contributing factor to the development of band erosion. The popularization of the pars flaccida approach over the perigastric technique not only decreased the incidence of prolapse but also eliminated the need for operative dissection directly adjacent to the gastric serosa. By avoiding dissection close to the gastric wall, the pars flaccida approach is favored over the perigastric technique. The increased dissection in and around the gastric serosal typical of the perigastric approach may have

Table 28.1. Incidence of erosion of Lap Band System in various studies.

FDA trial—Bioenterics	$n = 299$	1%
Bellachew et al.	$n = 763$	0.9%
Cadiere et al.	$n = 652$	0.3%
Favretti et al.	$n = 830$	0.5%
Fielding et al.	$n = 335$	0%
Vertruyen et al.	$n = 543$	1%

contributed to microinjuries of the gastric wall and eventual erosion. In cases in which esophageal injury or gastric perforation is suspected, the surgical injury should be definitively addressed and surgeons should strongly consider abandoning placement of the adjustable gastric band until a later date. A significant percentage of band erosions are clinically silent and chronic, occurring generally slowly and undetected until discovered incidentally during upper endoscopy.

The typical clinical course for band erosion is one of slow penetration into the gastric lumen. As this process can take months and even years to develop, the band has had adequate time to develop a protective peritoneal layer covering the band and its attached tubing, protecting the patient from peritonitis and abdominal sepsis. The slow leakage of gastric secretions into and around the band provokes a chronic irritation, preventing spontaneous healing. Small undetected microerosions develop into larger erosions. Symptoms may be absent until tracking of gastric contents along the band tubing reaches the subcutaneous tissue in and around the port. The peritonealized connecting tubing provides a conduit from the site of erosion to the subcutaneous port, resulting in drainage of gastric secretions and bacteria directly to the port site. The relatively poor immunologic ability of the subcutaneous layer of fat to adequately handle the presence of even small amounts of gastric secretions results in a chronic inflammatory irritation. Eventually this inflammatory irritation results in a clinically obvious port site infection and often presents as wound breakdown and exposure of the subcutaneous port. For the majority of cases, the first clinical sign that erosion has occurred is the development of an unexpected and unexplained port site infection. Initial treatments of drainage and antibiotics are not successful.

Alternatively, the development of gastric ulcers may lead to erosions and, as a result, routine over-the-counter nonsteroidal anti-inflammatory drug (NSAID) use should be discouraged in order to decrease the possible development of gastric erosion. Patients with debilitating arthritis are often dependent on NSAID use and can be managed more judiciously with prescription NSAIDs or Cox-II inhibitors as a preferred anti-inflammatory medication. Postoperative visits should include a history as to the use of NSAIDs, and particular attention should be paid to those patients using large or routine over-the-counter NSAIDs. Although NSAID use is not predictive of the development of band erosion, the use of routine NSAIDs should be monitored and restricted to those patients with a true need for these medications.

Because the onset of gastric erosion can be silent and take years to develop, some patients may present with unexplained failure of the restrictive mechanism and what appears to be a nonfunctioning band. Many of these patients have a history of good weight loss and adequate satiety with good satisfaction. Unexplained failure to lose weight or the development of weight gain accompanied with the inability to regulate the stoma with percutaneous adjustments should raise the suspicion of band erosion. In cases of unexplained loss of restriction despite adequate adjustments, postoperative endoscopy provides definitive diagnosis of the presence of gastric erosion.

Band erosion occurs at a higher rate in those patients who have undergone repositioning or replacement of their initial band, or who have had band placement following previous bariatric or gastric procedures.

C. Diagnosis

The clinical manifestations of band erosion can be diverse. The most common presenting symptom is unexplained infection at the port site. A review of 1,497 consecutive lap band patients discovered 17 erosions. Clinical manifestations of erosion included port site abscess in 40.6% of patients, port site sinus in 11.6%, subphrenic abscess in 11.6%, unexplained weight gain in 11.6%, left pyelonephritis in 5.8%, band deflation in 5.8%, peritonitis in 5.8%, and mucous collection at the port site in 5.8% (Figs. 28.1 and 28.2).

Upper GI endoscopy provides the most definitive evidence of band erosion. Endoscopic examination by the operative surgeons or by a gastroenterologist familiar with the device is preferred. Most erosions occur between the gastric fundus anteriorly and the band at the location where the fundus has been used to plicate or cover the portion of the band lateral to the buckle. Endoscopic examination with a

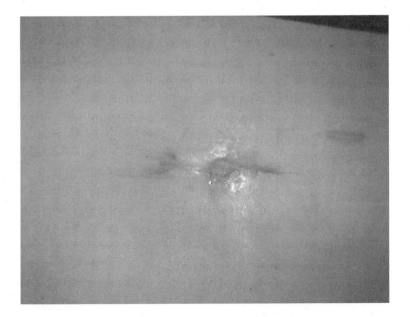

Figure 28.1. Typical nonhealing port site infection.

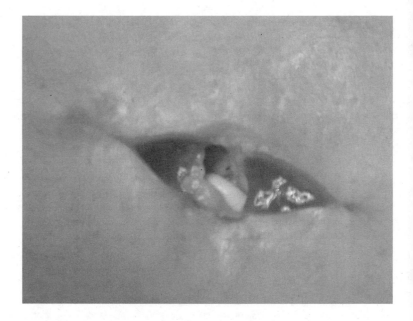

Figure 28.2. Opened chronically infected port site. Tubing is visible within established sinus tract.

retroflexed view of the band deformity and careful examination for the presence of visible sutures or visible band material is essential to avoid missing the diagnosis of band erosion. It is surprisingly easy to miss small erosions, as the erosion can be hidden under the deformity caused by a properly positioned band device. Meticulous and careful examination using the retroflexed view of the entire deformity caused by the band device is essential (Fig. 28.3).

In cases in which no erosion is identified despite adequate endoscopic examination, repeat endoscopic examination should be considered. Follow-up endoscopic examination should be considered within 6 months following the initial endoscopy to confirm the absence of erosion (Figs. 28.4 and 28.5).

Upper GI swallow and gastric imaging studies are rarely helpful in establishing the diagnosis of gastric erosion. Except for rare cases in which the band migrates intraluminally, these imaging studies will typically reveal normal band position and normal flow through band. The principal study used to establish the diagnosis of band erosion is direct examination via upper GI flexible endoscopic examination.

D. Treatment and Postoperative Course

Once the diagnosis of band erosion has been established, the treatment should be band removal. Removal of the device is typically performed laparoscopically, although there are reports of the band being removed endoscopically.

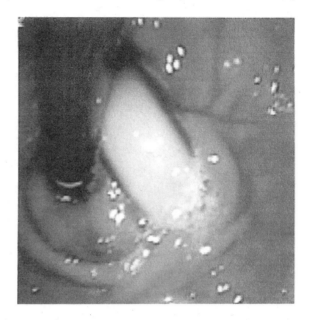

Figure 28.3. Eroded Lap Band, retroflexed view. Note that the endoscope does not pass within the ring of the device as a result the band is nonfunctional and creates no restrictive mechanism.

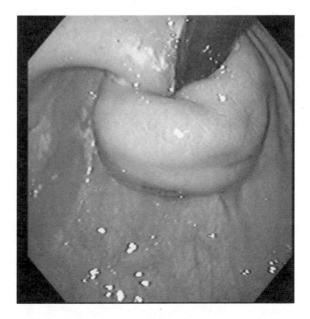

Figure 28.4. Subtle erosion barely visible except for hint of suture material.

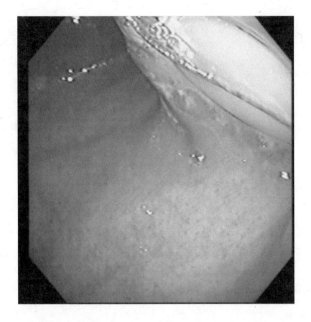

Figure 28.5. Same erosion as in Fig. 28.4, but with different endoscopic view reveals large visible erosion.

Supporters of endoscopic removal advocate waiting until intragastric migration of the band has occurred in order to remove the device endoscopically. Intragastric migration of the band is not a common event and the degree of erosion is not extensive enough to allow successful endoscopic removal of the device in most patients. The overwhelming majority of patients will benefit from removal of eroded devices laparoscopically without unnecessary delay. Furthermore, the endoscopic removal of an eroded represents an advanced procedure which requires specialized instrumentation and experience. The recommended technique for most erosions encountered will be to utilize a laparoscopic approach to explant the eroded device.

The steps of laparoscopic removal of an eroded adjustable gastric band are as follows:

1.   Identification of the lap band tubing
2.   Localization of the adjustable gastric band buckle and transaction of the band
3.   Identification and closure of the gastric erosion
4.   Drainage of the site with a closed system drain

Laparoscopic removal of an eroded adjustable gastric band is a challenging procedure. It is common to find dense and tenacious adhesions between the omentum and abdominal wall, as well as between the left lobe of the liver and the anterior gastric wall. In order to remove the device safely and minimize operative dissection, identification and location of the band tubing are essential. The tubing is typically encased with surrounding omentum and can be difficult to localize. Once identified, the tubing can be transected and used as a guide to direct the operative dissection directly to the buckle of the adjustable gastric band. It is common to discover a severe inflammatory reaction along the stomach wall adjoining the left lobe of the liver. These adhesions can be difficult to dissect but are progressively released, using the tubing as a guide until the cuff or buckle of the band is exposed and transected which allows easy removal of the device. Limited dissection in and around the buckle in order to free the buckle from surrounding tissue is all that is necessary to allow safe removal of the eroded band. There is no need to take down the gastric plication, and this excessive surgical dissection is discouraged. Once transected, the band can be easily removed by slipping it out from its perigastric position and removing it from the abdomen (Figs. 28.6 and 28.7).

The remaining gastric perforation should be located and closed. If possible, the defect is sutured in two layers and then evaluated for leaks. Installation of methylene blue dye mixed into a liter of saline into the gastric lumen by the anesthesiologist is sufficient to identify any leakage at the site of the erosion. If identified, the site of the leakage should be closed with endoscopic sutures. Additional inflammatory processes such as subphrenic abscess are relatively uncommon but, if present, should be drained. Drainage of the area with a closed drain should be performed to control any leakage that might develop postoperatively.

The postoperative course following removal of an eroded band should be unremarkable. A postoperative upper GI swallow is performed to rule out persistent

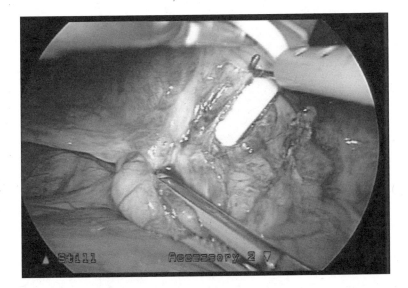

Figure 28.6. Dissection of eroded Lap Band buckle using tubing as a guide.

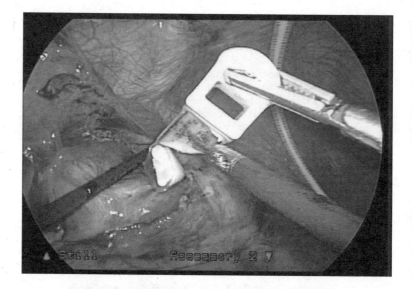

Figure 28.7. Transection and removal of the eroded band.

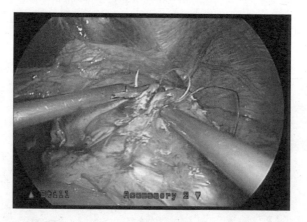

Figure 28.8. Oversewing of site of gastric perforation.

leakage from the erosion site and allow removal of the drain on the first post-operative day. Most patients can be discharged on their first postoperative day and diet can be resumed. We typically keep patients on a liquid diet for the first 5 days following band removal before beginning to advance their diet. Removal of an eroded band is a well-tolerated procedure and rarely develops postoperative complications. Infectious complications are rare. Patients are maintained on postoperative antibiotics for several days following band removal.

Although it is possible to replace an eroded band with a new replacement band simultaneously at the time of band removal, it is not a recommended practice. Most authors support addressing the issue in a delayed approach, postponing any consideration for band replacement or conversion to an alternative bariatric procedure for at least several months. Alternative bariatric procedures or band replacement can be considered at a later date and individualized for the specific needs of the individual patient.

E. Summary

Adjustable gastric band erosion is a rare complication, affecting fewer than 1% of patients undergoing this procedure. Erosion should be suspected in patients exhibiting signs of port site infection, unexplained loss of satiety, and nonfunctioning bands. The diagnosis is made endoscopically at the time of upper GI endoscopy, and requires careful endoscopic examination of the area.

Erosions can be classified as occurring early and late. The mechanism of early erosion is most likely secondary to surgical trauma resulting in partial thickness injury of the gastric serosa. The presence of the foreign body allows for injury to continue. Band pressure and ischemia secondary to percutaneous adjustment may play a role in promoting development of these partial thickness injuries into full-thickness erosions. Aggressive postoperative adjustments may play a further role in promoting gastric ischemia in the areas around the band, although this has yet to be proved to be a contributing factor in band erosion. Erosions that occur late are thought to develop as a result of multiple factors; smoking, NSAID use, excessive operative dissection, and postoperative ischemia, as well as tight gastric plication, have all been postulated as causes for postoperative erosion. Previous bariatric and gastric procedures such as Nissen fundoplication may contribute to ischemia at the operative site and enhance the development of gastric erosion. The role of pressure necrosis following band adjustment has not been directly associated with the development of late erosions. Judicious use of postoperative adjustments and avoiding the temptation to perform a "large fill" may be beneficial in decreasing the possible association of pressure necrosis and band erosion.

Erosion is rarely a surgical emergency and treatment can be deferred and scheduled electively. Definitive treatment of gastric erosion is band removal and can be accomplished laparoscopically in nearly every case, with most patients discharged less than 24 hours after admission.

F. Selected References

Abu-Abeid S, Keidar A, Gavert N, et al. The clinical spectrum of band erosion following laparoscopic adjustable silicone gastric banding for morbid obesity. Surg Endosc 2003;17: 861–863.

Belachew M, Belva PH, Desaive C. Long-term results of laparoscopic adjustable gastric banding for the treatment of morbid obesity. Obes Surg 2002;12:564–568.

Belachew M, Legrand MJ, Defechereux TH, et al. Laparoscopic adjustable silicone gastric banding in the treatment of morbid obesity: a preliminary report. Surg Endosc 1994;81354–1365.

Cadiere GB, Himpens J, Vertruyen M, et al. Laparoscopic gastroplasty (adjustable silicone gastric banding). Semin Laparosc Surg 2000;7:55–65.

Dargent J. Laparoscopic adjustable gastric banding: lessons from the first 500 patients in a single institution. Obes Surg 1999;9:446–452.

Favretti F, Cadiere G B, Segato G, et al. Lap-Band for the treatment of morbid obesity: a 6-year experience of 509 patients. Obes Surg 1999;9:327–329.

Favretti F, Cadiere GB, Segato G, et al. Laparoscopic banding: selection and technique in 830 patients. Obes Surg 2002;12:385–390.

Fielding GA, Rhodes M, Nathanson LK. Laparoscopic gastric banding for morbid obesity: surgical outcome in 335 cases. Surg Endosc 1999;13:550–554.

Meir E, Van Baden M. Adjustable silicone gastric banding and band erosion: personal experience and hypotheses. Obes Surg 1999;9:191–193.

Szold A, Abu-Abeid S. Laparoscopic adjustable silicone gastric banding for morbid obesity: results and complications in 715 patients. Surg Endosc 2002;16:230–233.

US Food and Drug Administration, Center for Devices and Radiological Health. LAP-BAND Adjustable Gastric Banding (LAGB) System—P000008. Available at http://www.fda.gov/cdrh/pdf/p000008.htm. Accessed August 23, 2002.

Vertruyen M. Experience with LAP-BAND system up to 7 years. Obes Surg 2002;12:5 69–572.

Weiner R, Wagner D, Bockhorn H. Laparoscopic gastric banding for morbid obesity. J Laparoendosc Adv Surg Technique 1999;9:23–30.

Weiss H, Nehoda H, Labeck B, et al. Gastroscopic band removal after intragastric migration of adjustable gastric band: a new minimal invasive technique. Obes Surg 2000;10:167–170.

V. Guidelines and Accreditation in Bariatric Surgery

29. Society of American Gastrointestinal and Endoscopic Surgeons (SAGES) Bariatric Credentialing Guidelines

Shawn Tsuda and Daniel B. Jones

A. Introduction

With the continued growth of bariatric surgery, there has been scrutiny of outcomes. Professional societies, insurance companies, and watch-dog organizations have developed guidelines for the best practices of bariatric surgery and the granting of privileges to qualified surgeons to perform bariatric procedures.

The Society of American Gastrointestinal and Endoscopic Surgeons (SAGES) has a history of authoring privileging and practice guidelines for the promotion of patient safety and improvement of clinical outcomes. Currently, there are 15 such guidelines, ranging from the granting of privileges for gastrointestinal endoscopy to the use of deep venous thrombosis prophylaxis in laparoscopic surgery.

In July 2003, the Board of Governors of SAGES approved the Guidelines for Institutions Granting Bariatric Privileges Utilizing Laparoscopic Techniques. The statement was originally prepared jointly with members of the American Society of Bariatric Surgery (ASBS), now the American Society of Metabolic and Bariatric Surgery (ASMBS). Since then, the ASMBS has published its own guidelines on the granting of privileges for bariatric procedures.

B. The SAGES Guidelines for Institutions Granting Bariatric Privileges Utilizing Laparoscopic Techniques

In the SAGES guideline for the clinical application of laparoscopic bariatric surgery, which was published concurrently with its privileging guidelines, laparoscopic as well as open weight loss procedures were established as durable treatments for morbid obesity as long as practiced by appropriately trained surgical teams within programs that provide perioperative and long-term management. The indications for weight loss surgery were derived from the 1991 National Institutes of Health Consensus Conference for the surgical management of morbidly obese patients. More recently, the

2003 SAGES Appropriateness Conference restated the appropriateness of duodenal switch, banded gastroplasty, laparoscopic adjustable band, and laparoscopic gastric bypass based on current evidence. The *SAGES Guidelines for Institutions Granting Bariatric Privileges Utilizing Laparoscopic Techniques* addresses who should perform bariatric procedures by stating the purpose, definitions, training requirements, institutional support, and maintenance of privileges that would facilitate local hospital staffs to ensure high quality care with a systems-based approach.

1. Purpose

SAGES recommends that their guidelines be used by health care institutions and hospital administrations as an adjunct to the Joint Commission on Accreditation of Healthcare Organizations (JCAHO) to implement privileges for bariatric surgery. In contrast to guidelines developed by the Betsy Lehman Center, ASMBS, and ACS, which establish volume criteria for privileging that range between 25 and 50 weight loss procedures, SAGES states that the decision to grant privileges should *not* be based solely on the number of procedures performed. SAGES places the actual privileging structure on individual institutions, through a process that begins with the chief of surgery and is approved by a committee, board, or other governing body.

2. Definitions

The SAGES guidelines for bariatric privileging establishes nomenclature for mandatory recommendation (MUST/SHALL), highly desirable recommendation (SHOULD), optional recommendations (MAY/COULD), documentation of training, privileging, credentialing, competence, complete procedural conduct (ability to perform the operation from patient selection to open conversion if required), laparoscopy, types of bariatric procedures, and what constitutes a formal course of training.

As stated, SAGES places the adequacy (volume number) of the surgeon's experience on the individual institutions or the chief of surgery. Formal residency and/or fellowship training should be structured, but case numbers are not specified. For surgeons without formal training, preceptorship/proctorship and formal courses are offered as alternatives. A preceptor or proctor should be determined by the institution, be familiar with all aspects of the procedure, including patient selection, and be chosen in an unbiased, confidential, and objective manner. A formal course is not offered as adequate training to perform a procedure independently, but *should* be done for procedures for which privileges are being sought. Such courses must meet category 1 Continuing Medical Education requirements, include didactics by qualified surgeons, and involve hands-on experience with animate and/or inanimate models. Adjunctive aids include video reviews or computer programs. Examples are the SAGES Grand Rounds DVD for bariatric surgery or the SAGES *Pearls* series for laparoscopic Roux-en-Y gastric bypass.

C. Minimum Requirements for Privileging of Bariatric Procedures

The recommended mandatory requirements by SAGES consist of: (1) formal residency training in general surgery within an accredited program with subsequent certification by the American Board of Surgery if required by the institution; and (2) documentation that there exists adequate follow-up of patients, including nursing care, dietary care, counseling, support groups, exercise training, psychological care if needed, and a method of identifying and managing complications.

If the surgeon has formal training only in open bariatric surgery, SAGES recommends having a second surgeon who is trained in laparoscopic bariatric surgery, and is therefore complementary to their expertise. Alternatively, the surgeon may participate in a proctored experience deemed adequate by the chief of surgery.

If the surgeon has documented formal training in laparoscopic bariatric surgery, SAGES recommends that the volume of open and laparoscopic cases be demonstrated for the type of procedures to be done, and that a complementary surgeon experienced in open procedures be available if needed. The adequacy of case volume/experience is to be determined by the chief of surgery.

If the surgeon has no documented formal residency training in either laparoscopic open bariatric surgery, they are expected to take a formal course AND be proctored by a qualified surgeon who is approved by the institution of practice.

D. Institutional Support

Adequate equipment and staff training are expected to be in place prior to starting a bariatric program. Two skilled surgeons are recommended for laparoscopic bariatric procedures, or a surgeon and a skilled first assistant.

E. Maintenance of Privileges

SAGES recommends that the chief of surgery or appropriate institutional body should determine the criteria for provisional privileges, monitoring of performance and outcomes, and continuing education requirements (meetings and courses). The guideline states that outcome data should be reviewed after 6 months of the granting of privileges, and regularly thereafter as compared with published national benchmarks. Any denial of privileges should have an appeal process in place.

F. Selected References

ASBS Bariatric Training Committee. American Society for Bariatric Surgery Guidelines for Granting Privileges in Bariatric Surgery. Surg Obes Rel Dis 2006;2(1):65–67.

Bessler M, Champion K, Cohen R, et al. Laparoscopic Roux-en-Y gastric bypass: SAGES pearls. Cine-Med 2005.

Gagner M, Ren C, Flum D, et al. SAGES grand rounds: bariatric Surgery. CineMed. 2007.

Guidelines for the Clinical Application of Laparoscopic Bariatric Surgery. http://www.sages.org/sagespublicationprint.php?doc=30. Accessed June 25,2006.

Jones DB, DeMaria E, Provost DA, et al. Optimal management of the morbidly obese patient: SAGES appropriateness conference statement. Surg Endosc 2004;18(7):1029–1037.

Kelly J, Shikora S, Jones DB, et al. Best practice updates for surgical care in weight loss surgery. Obes Res 2007; in press.

SAGES. Guidelines for institutions granting bariatric privileges utilizing laparoscopic techniques. Surg Endosc 2003;17:2037–2040.

Schirmer B, Jones DB. American College of Surgeons Bariatric Surgery Center Network. ACS Bull 2007;92(8):21–27.

Schirmer BD, Schauer PR, Flum DR, et al. Bariatric surgery training: getting your ticket punched. J Gastrointe Surg 2007;11:807–812.

30. Reporting of Bariatric Surgery Outcomes

Gavitt A. Woodard and John M. Morton

A. Introduction

Morbid obesity is rapidly increasing globally and is the leading cause of preventable cause of death in the United States. The only effective and enduring treatment for morbid obesity remains bariatric surgery. Both the growth in the prevalence of obesity and the success of weight loss surgery has led to truly spectacular growth in utilization of bariatric surgery. Outcomes have driven both the rise and fall of bariatric surgery over time. A clear reason for the recent growth of bariatric surgery was the 2004 approval of weight loss surgery by the Centers for Medicare and Medicaid Services, which was driven by outcomes studies. In the 1970s, serious adverse outcomes associated with jejunal-ileal bypass led to its ultimate demise, uniquely becoming the only operation to be banned by the FDA. Currently, both strong consumer and insurer interest in weight loss surgery and increased societal awareness of patient safety have directed intense interest in the outcomes of bariatric surgery. Standardization of outcomes reporting in bariatric surgery has long been an issue of contention; however, recent events have demonstrated that bariatric surgery is entering a watershed in outcomes reporting.

B. Outcomes Definitions

Defining the problem of obesity and its current solution of surgery is paramount. Obesity is currently defined by the National Heart, Lung, and Blood Institute as body mass index (BMI) in four classes: (I) 30–35, (II) 35–40, (III) 40–50, and (IV) >50. BMI has been clearly recognized as the best measure of obesity, surpassing cumbersome measurements such as fat content, waist/hip circumference, or percent of weight over ideal weight. Anthropometric measurements have the disadvantage of recorder variability while ideal weight provides an elusive definition. BMI has strong correlation to certain diseases such as type 2 diabetes. In fact, BMI alone may be sufficient in documenting the presence of insulin resistance and metabolic syndrome instead of using the ATP III criteria. By using BMI as a marker for obesity, the Centers for Disease Control have documented a phenomenal growth in obesity in the United States.

Correspondingly, weight loss surgery has grown in response to this public health concern. Since 1997, bariatric surgery in the United States has grown sevenfold, with gastric bypass remaining the most common procedure. In the remainder of the world, adjustable gastric banding is the leading weight loss surgery. Defining these weight loss procedures appears straightforward, with each falling into the realms of restrictive, malabsorptive, or a combination of the two. These general categories will most likely be amended with the advent of new technology, such as vagal nerve stimulation or NOTES procedures. Prospectively maintained databases for new technologies or procedures such as the NOSCAR database will allow for better recognition of efficacy and safety for these procedures. Furthermore, even well-established procedures such as gastric bypass have significant variation, which may render comparisons tenuous. For example, a gastric bypass has several points of disparity, such as open vs. laparoscopic, antecolic vs. retrocolic, sparing of vagal branches, limb length, etc. The landmark 1991 National Institutes of Health (NIH) Consensus Conference recognized some of these inherent difficulties when they wrote, "One of the key problems in the current reports of case series in surgical therapy is the lack of standards for comparison."

C. Data Sources

Many efforts have been made to collect data for bariatric surgery through individual surgeons, surgical societies, or research initiatives, including the International Bariatric Surgery Registry, Society for Advanced Gastrointestinal Endoscopic Surgery (SAGES) Outcomes Initiative, Swedish Obese Subjects Trial, and the ongoing NIH Longitudinal Assessment of Bariatric Surgery (LABS) trial. Bariatric surgery outcomes have also been reported from existing administrative claims data, such as Medicare, Nationwide In-Patient Sample (NIS), and University Health Consortium (UHC).

A PubMed query including the search terms of surgery, weight loss, and outcomes yielded 465 results. Evaluation of these different data sources should rest on evidence-based criteria. For example, prospective, clinically derived data through standardized definitions are clearly ideal. However, prospective data take time to collect and emerging trends of care may not be scrutinized until deleterious effects have already taken place. Administrative claims data, such as exists in Medicare, NIS, or UHC, provide the advantage of easily obtainable data in large numbers that are multi-institutional. In addition, for certain rare procedures, such as adolescent bariatric surgery, administrative databases may be the only means of determining procedure trends in sizable numbers. Administrative, claims data certainly supports the proverb, "You search where there is light." However, these databases can provide conflicting results. These data are not obtained for clinical practice but for billing purposes. The clear shortcomings of administrative claims data are that they are deficient in clinical data, such as BMI, which are integral for risk adjustment. Administrative claims data do render the essential function of "a canary in a coal mine." While these claims data do not always render a definitive conclusion, they can serve as an early warning system regarding emerging trends in practice patterns and outcomes.

D. Center of Excellence Movement

The influence of administrative claims data was clearly seen with the 2005 study which found a 1-year 4.6% all-cause mortality rate for Medicare patients undergoing gastric bypass. The study had the advantages of being multi-institutional and having large numbers; however, it lacked robust risk adjustment, applicability of results to the general gastric bypass population, and specificity of cause of death. Despite those limitations, it did demonstrate an important association between surgeon volume and outcomes. These results of higher than expected mortality and positive volume-outcome correlation led to the Centers of Medicare and Medicaid Services (CMMS) mandating two requirements: a prohibition of gastric bypass in Medicare recipients over 65 years of age and an obligation that weight loss surgery be performed at high-volume Centers of Excellence (COE) as defined by the two certifying bodies of the American Society of Bariatric and Metabolic Surgery (ASMBS) and American College of Surgeons (ACS). While the prohibition of weight loss surgery in Medicare recipients has been overturned, the Center of Excellence initiative has remained in force and gathered strength. Many other payers have followed CMMS's lead in requiring that weight loss surgery be performed by high-volume surgeons, leading to a preponderance of gastric bypass procedures being performed in high-volume centers. With the advent of the ASMBS and ACS databases, bariatric surgery has entered a new era in outcomes reporting. As the official databases for bariatric surgery, there is a heightened interest in the cost and components of the databases as well as a hope that a single standard will be achieved.

One constant in data collection is change. All databases should be organic enough to either grow or diminish over time. There is an essential creative tension in outcomes collection between the desire for covering every aspect of data and the need for brevity to ensure completion of data. A bariatric surgery database should have ideal components and means of collection. Ideally, the data should be collected prospectively and audited by trained clinicians with standardized definitions entered via the web to allow for ease and speed of entry. Clearly, these means of data collection are costly and cannot be borne by the individual surgeon but should be a hospital-based responsibility to achieve and maintain COE status.

E. Ideal Bariatric Surgery Database

An ideal bariatric surgery database should include the following: patient demographics, hospital characteristics, surgical outcomes, and long-term follow-up. Patient demographics include age, gender, BMI, comorbidities, functional status, quality of life, and socioeconomic status. As mentioned, BMI appears to be a sufficient measure for weight and avoids the variety of reporting currently seen for ideal body weight. A study by Dixon found a tremendous lack of standardization for ideal weight. However, BMI may not be appropriate in the adolescent population, in which growth in height is expected and age percentile of weight would be more appropriate. A clear standard for weight loss needs to be set and should not be based on ideal weight given the elusiveness of that ideal.

Comorbidity definition and documentation are essential for both risk adjustment of outcomes as well as accurate assessment of resolution. The effects of morbid obesity upon body systems are legion and profound. Ali and colleagues performed a detailed taxonomy of the common comorbidities associated with obesity that may serve as an ideal comorbidity scale to embrace. Some comorbidities may defy succinct or concrete definition such as musculoskeletal impairment, whereas others such as lipid abnormalities have clear consensus. It has been demonstrated that obesity is an inflammatory disease and that inflammation markers such as high-sensitivity C-reactive protein improve dramatically after surgery. As result, clinically defined comorbidities may be used in conjunction with biochemical markers to fully define the penumbra of obesity-related diseases.

Furthermore, hospital characteristics should be described in the classic Donabedian model of quality: structure, process, and outcomes. The structural measures of bariatric surgery quality should include the following: Center of Excellence designation, volume of procedures performed, fellowship-trained bariatric surgeons, and multidisciplinary specialists in anesthesia, gastroenterology, nutrition, and psychology. **Process measure**s of bariatric surgery quality might include adherence to Surgery Care Improvement Project (SCIP) measures, selective use of IVC filters, and clinical pathways. Finally, **outcomes measures** of quality may include weight loss, morbidity including reoperations/readmissions, and mortality. Mortality should be represented as 30 day, 90 day, 1 year, and 5 year to fully comprehend the impact of weight loss surgery upon survival. A telling point in the land mark Adams' Utah study on gastric bypass and survival demonstrated that the risk of mortality by maintaining a morbidly obese status in the control group was *equivalent* to the mortality risk of surgery in the first year.

F. Outcomes: Weight Loss

The degree of weight loss associated with bariatric surgery is dependent upon which operation is employed. Recently, several studies have provided considerable information regarding weight loss after surgery. In the Swedish Obese Subjects Study, which compared medically and surgically treated obese patients, there were striking differences between the two groups regarding weight loss. At 10 years the conventionally treated group had a 1.6% increase in total weight, while the surgically treated group saw a 24% decrease in total weight. Among the different surgical procedures performed in the Swedish Obese Subjects (SOS) Study, the highest amount of total weight loss was for gastric bypass (25%), followed by vertical banded gastroplasty (17%), and adjustable gastric banding (13%).

Two important studies have reviewed the entire published medical literature regarding bariatric surgery. These two meta-analyses provide strong validation for the efficacy of weight loss surgery. The outcomes after surgically induced weight loss published in the last years are impressive. The meta-analysis by Buchwald found that the degree of weight loss is lowest for restrictive procedures and highest for malabsorptive procedures. In this meta-analysis of 22,094 patients (mean age: 47 years, mean BMI 46.9, 72.6 % women), the mean percentage of excess weight loss was 61.2% for all patients. Excessive weight loss was higher for patients who underwent for gastric bypass (61.6%) or gastroplasty

(68.2%) compared with those who received gastric banding (47.5%). Similar results for weight loss were reported by Maggard in the *Annals of Internal Medicine*. In this study, weight loss in kilograms for at least 3 years postoperatively was as follows: gastric banding (35 kg), gastroplasty (32 kg), biliopancreatic diversion/duodenal switch (53 kg), and gastric bypass (42 kg).

G. Outcomes: Comorbidity Resolution

Weight loss surgery is a singular medical intervention that has the unique ability to reverse or improve the numerous medical conditions associated with obesity. The leading cause of death in the United States remains heart disease and stroke, with 300,000 patients dying annually. The primary medical conditions contributing to this devastating human toll are diabetes, hypertension, and hyperlipidemia. These three comorbidities, along with visceral obesity, constitute the metabolic syndrome that is a strong risk factor for cardiovascular mortality. All three of these cardiovascular risk factors improved as described in an important *Annals of Surgery* publication by Schauer et al. regarding laparoscopic gastric bypass with the following resolution rates: diabetes (82%), hypertension (70%), and hyperlipidemia (63%).

The SOS study provided further demonstration of the ameliorative effect of bariatric surgery. At 10 years in the SOS study, surgically treated obese patients had substantial improvements in their cardiac risk factors, in comparison with nonsurgically treated obese patients. Surgically treated obese patients had 25% reduction in hypertension, 43% improvement in HDL, and 75% reduction in diabetes in comparison with the medically treated group. Another study found clear, consistent, and convincing resolution of every conventional risk factor at 1 year after gastric bypass surgery.

Gastric bypass has assembled the most evidence for resolution of comorbidities. However, all weight loss surgeries promote resolution of these important medical problems. Each procedure has a different degree of improvement for different comorbidities as demonstrated by the *JAMA* article by Buchwald. For diabetes, each procedure has the following resolution rate: banding (48%), gastroplasty (68%), gastric bypass (84%), and biliopancreatic diversion/duodenal switch (98%). Hyperlipidemia is another cardiac risk factor that is improved by each weight loss surgery by different amounts: banding (71%), gastroplasty (81%), gastric bypass (94%), and biliopancreatic diversion/duodenal switch (99%). Finally, hypertension is also resolved by the following procedures at the accompanying rates: banding (38%), gastroplasty (73%), gastric bypass (75%), and biliopancreatic diversion/duodenal switch (81%).

Beyond the tremendous improvement in cardiac risk factors, weight loss surgery also provides enormous enhancement of the myriad medical problems that obesity engenders. An important health concern associated with obesity is sleep apnea, which carries significant health risks, including premature death. Fortunately, weight loss surgery also improves sleep apnea as demonstrated by Buchwald: banding (95%), gastroplasty (77%), gastric bypass (87%), and biliopancreatic diversion/duodenal switch (95%). Joint disease is a leading health concern that severely decreases both personal satisfaction and work productivity. Schauer demonstrated 88% resolution or improvement of joint disease for morbidly obese patients undergoing laparoscopic gastric bypass.

In addition, the leading digestive health complaint, gastroesophageal reflux disease, is cured or improved at a 96% rate. The most prevalent liver disease, nonalcoholic fatty liver disease, is very commonly associated with morbid obesity and is also very often improved by weight loss surgery.

Furthermore, weight loss surgery has been demonstrated to either eliminate or improve the following health conditions: venous stasis disease, gout, asthma, psuedotumor cerebri, urinary incontinence, and infertility.[32]

H. Outcomes: Quality of Life

Quality of life in the morbidly obese patient is clearly diminished due to self-image, economic discrimination, lack of medical access, and societal lack of acceptance. Of note, weight loss surgery is also equally powerful in reversing poor quality of life as it is in resolving medical problems. There is ample evidence to demonstrate improvement in quality of life after weight loss surgery. The most accepted survey in medicine for quality of life is the SF36, which has been demonstrated to improve sharply after bariatric surgery. Also, disease-specific quality of life instruments have also shown improvement after surgery. Finally, depression is a disease that can severely impair quality of life. A measure of depression, Beck Depression Index, has been demonstrated to decline by half following weight loss surgery.

I. Outcomes: Cost-Effectiveness

Given the dramatic effects upon comorbidities that bariatric surgery renders, it is apparent that bariatric surgery can also provide reduction in health care costs. This reduction in health care costs has been demonstrated in the province of Quebec, where surgically treated patients incurred $CN6,000 less in health care costs versus morbidly obese patients treated nonsurgically. Two cost-effectiveness analyses demonstrated that bariatric surgery is a dominant strategy with a range of $5,000 to $35,600 per Quality Adjusted Life Year (QALY). Both studies show that bariatric surgery provides a QALY at lower rate than $50,000, the common marker of cost-effectiveness.

J. Outcomes: Survival

Weight loss and comorbidity resolution each contribute to increased survival for the surgically treated morbidly obese patient. Several studies have demonstrated improved survival after gastric bypass surgery. Flum et al. noted a 33% reduction in mortality for morbidly obese patients who underwent surgery versus morbidly obese patients who were treated medically. McDonald et al. also provided clear evidence for a survival benefit in the surgically treated morbidly obese patient. This retrospective analysis of type 2 diabetic patients with morbid obesity, who underwent either gastric bypass operation or did not undergo surgery, demonstrated a mortality rate of only 9% in the surgical group during the 9-year follow-up compared with 28% in the nonsurgical control group. A decisive conclusion regarding the survival benefit conferred by gastric bypass surgery is provided by a population-based study from Quebec, Canada. The mortality rate in the bariatric surgery cohort was 0.68% compared with 6.17% in controls, which translated to a tremendous 89% reduction in the relative risk of death.

Finally, two recent articles in the *New England Journal of Medicine* conclusively demonstrated the survival benefit engendered by bariatric surgery. Sjostrom and colleagues found in the SOS trial, a hazard ratio of 0.71 demonstrating a reduction in mortality for surgically treated morbidly obese patients versus controls. The SOS incorporated three different surgical techniques provided 10-year follow-up data. Adams et al. also showed a decided survival benefit after gastric bypass surgery. From the state of Utah, 7,925 surgical patients and 7,925 severely obese control subjects were matched for age, sex, and body mass index. During a mean follow-up of 7 years, adjusted long-term mortality from any cause in the surgery group decreased by 40%, as compared with that in the control group. In addition, cause-specific mortality in the surgery group decreased by 56% for coronary artery disease, 92% for diabetes, and 60% for cancer. However, rates of death not caused by disease, such as accidents and suicide, were 58% higher in the surgery group than in the control group. This latter finding of increased deaths not caused by disease was not present in the SOS study, in which gastric bypass was not predominant. A common denominator to both accidents and suicides is alcohol abuse: It has been demonstrated that gastric bypass profoundly alters alcohol metabolism. There are clear and consistent data to support the fact that bariatric surgery renders a survival benefit to the morbidly obese patient.

K. Conclusions

While more work needs to be done with data collection, definitions, and standards, bariatric surgery is a sterling example of outcomes driven care. For the first time in US surgical history, the government mandated a level of performance for a surgical specialty. The bariatric surgery community met that challenge of federal oversight with enthusiasm and results. In a challenging population of patients with multiple medical problems, effective and enduring care is provided. Outcomes have demonstrated that in the right hands and in the right patients, bariatric surgery is a life-saving procedure.

L. Selected References

Adams TD, Gress RE, Smith SC, et al. Long-term mortality after gastric bypass surgery. NEJM 2007;357(8):753–761.

Alhassan S, Kiazand A, Balise RR, et al. Metabolic syndrome: do clinical criteria identify similar individuals among overweight premenopausal women? Metabolism 2008;57(1):49-56.

Ali MR, Maguire MB, Wolfe BM. Assessment of obesity-related comorbidities: a novel scheme for evaluating bariatric surgical patients. J Am Coll Surg 2006;202(1):70–77.

Belle SH, Berk PD, Courcoulas AP, et al. Safety and efficacy of bariatric surgery: longitudinal assessment of bariatric surgery. Surg Obes Relat Dis 2007;3(2):116–126.

Best M, Neuhauser D. Avedis Donabedian: father of quality assurance and poet. Qual Saf Health Care 2004;13(6):472–473.

Birkmeyer NJ, Wei Y, Goldfaden A, et al. Characteristics of hospitals performing bariatric surgery. JAMA 2006;295(3):282–284.

Bosy-Westphal A, Geisler C, Onur S, et al. Value of body fat mass vs anthropometric obesity indices in the assessment of metabolic risk factors. Int J Obes (Lond) 2006;30(3): 475–483.

Buchwald H, Williams SE. Bariatric surgery worldwide 2003. Obes Surg 2004;14(9): 1157–1164.

Buchwald H. The future of bariatric surgery. Obes Surg 2005;15(5):598–605.

Centers for Medicare and Medicaid Services. Decision memo for bariatric surgery for the treatment of morbid obesity (CAG-00250R). Available at http://www.cms.hhs.gov. Accessed February 2008.

Christou NV, Sampalis JS, Liberman M, et al. Surgery decreases long-term mortality, morbidity, and health care use in morbidly obese patients. Ann Surg 2004;240(3): 416–423; discussion 23–24.

Clegg A, Colquitt J, Sidhu M, et al. Clinical and cost effectiveness of surgery for morbid obesity: a systematic review and economic evaluation. Int J Obes Relat Metab Disord 2003;27(10):1167–1177.

Consensus Development Conference Panel. Gastrointestinal surgery for severe obesity. Ann Int Med 1991;115(12):956–961.

Craig BM, Tseng DS. Cost-effectiveness of gastric bypass for severe obesity. Am J Med 2002;113(6):491–498.

Dixon JB, Dixon ME, O'Brien PE. Depression in association with severe obesity: changes with weight loss. Arch Int Med 2003;163(17):2058–2065.

Dixon JB, McPhail T, O'Brien PE. Minimal reporting requirements for weight loss: current methods not ideal. Obes Surg 2005;15(7):1034–1039.

Dymek MP, Le Grange D, Neven K, et al. Quality of life after gastric bypass surgery: a cross-sectional study. Obes Res 2002;10(11):1135–1142.

Flum DR, Dellinger EP. Impact of gastric bypass operation on survival: a population-based analysis. J Am Coll Surg 2004;199(4):543–551.

Flum DR, Salem L, Elrod JA, et al. Early mortality among Medicare beneficiaries undergoing bariatric surgical procedures. JAMA 2005;294(15):1903–1908.

Griffen WO Jr, Young VL, Stevenson CC. A prospective comparison of gastric and jejunoileal bypass procedures for morbid obesity. Ann Surg 1977;186(4):500–509.

Hagedorn JC, Encarnacion B, Brat GA, et al. Does gastric bypass alter alcohol metabolism? Surg Obes Relat Dis 2007;3(5):543–548; discussion 8.

http://www.ncbi.nlm.nih.gov.laneproxy.stanford.edu/sites/entrez. Accessed April 12, 2008.

http://www.nhlbi.nih.gov/guidelines/obesity/ob_home.htm. Accessed April 12, 2008.

http://www.sages.org/projects/outcomes/index.php. Accessed April 12, 2008.

Klein S, Mittendorfer B, Eagon JC, et al. Gastric bypass surgery improves metabolic and hepatic abnormalities associated with nonalcoholic fatty liver disease. Gastroenterology 2006;130(6):1564–1572.

Lean ME, Powrie JK, Anderson AS, et al. Obesity, weight loss and prognosis in type 2 diabetes. Diabet Med 1990;7(3):228–233.

MacDonald KG Jr, Long SD, Swanson MS, et al. The gastric bypass operation reduces the progression and mortality of non-insulin-dependent diabetes mellitus. J Gastrointest Surg 1997;1(3):213–220; discussion 20.

Maggard MA, Shugarman LR, Suttorp M, et al. Meta-analysis: surgical treatment of obesity. Ann Intern Med 2005;142(7):547–559.

Nguyen NT, Goldman C, Rosenquist CJ, et al. Laparoscopic versus open gastric bypass: a randomized study of outcomes, quality of life, and costs. Ann Surg 2001;234(3): 279–289; discussion 89–91.

Nguyen NT, Morton JM, Wolfe BM, et al. The SAGES Bariatric Surgery Outcome Initiative. Surg Endosc 2005;19(11):1429–1438.

Ogden CL, Carroll MD, Curtin LR, et al. Prevalence of overweight and obesity in the United States, 1999-2004. JAMA 2006;295(13):1549–1555.

Pratt GM, McLees B, Pories WJ. The ASBS Bariatric Surgery Centers of Excellence program: a blueprint for quality improvement. Surg Obes Relat Dis 2006;2(5):497–503.

Russell TR. Yes, we can all get along: American College of Surgeons' response to editorial. Surg Obes Relat Dis 2006;2(5):567–568.

Sampalis JS, Liberman M, Auger S, et al. The impact of weight reduction surgery on health-care costs in morbidly obese patients. Obes Surg 2004;14(7):939–947.

Santry HP, Gillen DL, Lauderdale DS. Trends in bariatric surgical procedures. JAMA 2005;294(15):1909–1917.

Schauer PR, Ikramuddin S, Gourash W, et al. Outcomes after laparoscopic Roux-en-Y gastric bypass for morbid obesity. Ann Surg 2000;232(4):515–529.

Sjostrom L, Lindroos AK, Peltonen M, et al. Lifestyle, diabetes, and cardiovascular risk factors 10 years after bariatric surgery. NEJM 2004;351(26):2683–2693.

Sjostrom L, Narbro K, Sjostrom CD, et al. Effects of bariatric surgery on mortality in Swedish obese subjects. NEJM 2007;357(8):741–752.

Trus TL, Pope GD, Finlayson SR. National trends in utilization and outcomes of bariatric surgery. Surg Endosc 2005;19(5):616–620.

Varela JE, Hinojosa MW, Nguyen NT. Perioperative outcomes of bariatric surgery in adolescents compared with adults at academic medical centers. Surg Obes Relat Dis 2007;3(5):537–540; discussion 41–42.

Williams DB, Hagedorn JC, Lawson EH, et al. Gastric bypass reduces biochemical cardiac risk factors. Surg Obes Relat Dis 2007;3(1):8–13.

Wolfe BM, Morton JM. Weighing in on bariatric surgery: procedure use, readmission rates, and mortality. JAMA 2005;294(15):1960–1963.

Zhang W, Mason EE, Renquist KE, et al. Factors influencing survival following surgical treatment of obesity. Obes Surg 2005;15(1):43–50.

31. The Betsy Lehman Center Guidelines for Weight Loss Surgery

Matthew M. Hutter

A. Introduction

In 2003, as weight loss surgeries were being performed in increasing numbers, the media and public had significant concerns about the safety of these procedures. At that time, the Massachusetts Department of Public Health charged the Betsy Lehman Center for Patient Safety and Medical Error Reduction with the task of assessing weight loss surgery and developing evidence-based best practice recommendations for the safe and effective performance of these procedures. An expert panel on weight loss surgery was convened in 2004, and the resulting recommendations were published in *Obesity Research* in 2005. Three years later, the Betsy Lehman Center reconvened the Expert Panel on Weight Loss Surgery to update the initial recommendations based on the significant body of literature that had been published in the interim.

The best practice recommendations published by the Betsy Lehman Center have set the standard for weight loss surgery across the state of Massachusetts, and across the nation. The report was abstracted by the Agency for Healthcare Research and Quality (AHRQ) and adopted as the blueprint for the American College of Surgeons Bariatric Surgery Center Network accreditation program, which is recognized by the Centers for Medicare and Medicaid Services.

B. Methodology

The Betsy Lehman Center Expert Panel of Weight Loss Surgery consists of a multidisciplinary expert panel and 11 task groups. The expert panel and task groups were made up of members from all aspects of the care of the obese patient, including patients, surgeons, nurses, anesthetists, psychologists, psychiatrists, ethicists, nutritionists, internal medicine doctors, gastroenterologists, pediatricians, research methodologists, hospital administrators, as well as representatives from the insurers, Medicaid, the state board of registration in medicine, and the Department of Public Health.

A systematic review of the literature was performed, and relevant articles were abstracted using standardized data extraction tables. The available data were ranked according to levels of evidence based on study design (Table 31.1). Prospective, randomized controlled trials, or meta-analyses of such trials are

Table 31.1. Grading system for evidence-based recommendations.

Category A	Evidence obtained from at least one well-conducted randomized clinical trial or a systematic review of all relevant RCTs
Category B	Evidence from well-conducted prospective cohort studies, registry or meta-analysis of cohort studies, or population-based case-control studies
Category C	Evidence obtained from uncontrolled or poorly controlled clinical trials, or retrospective case-control analyses, cross-sectional studies, case series, or case reports
Category D	Evidence consisting of opinion from expert panels or the clinical experience of acknowledged authorities

Adapted from the criteria used by the US Preventive Services Task Force (USPSTF) and the American Diabetes Association.

given the highest level of evidence—Category A. Prospective cohort studies or case-control studies are considered Category B. Retrospective cohort studies or case series are considered Category C. For the areas in which there was no credible literature, recommendations were based on expert opinion—Category D.

All recommendations were vetted in an open forum, through a series of meetings, and edits were made until all recommendations were unanimously agreed upon by the expert panel in a formal voting process. Recommendations and supporting references were then published in a peer-reviewed journal.

C. Betsy Lehman I

Convened in 2004, the initial Betsy Lehman Center Expert Panel on Weight Loss Surgery consisted of 24 expert panel members and 9 task groups. Twelve articles were published in a special supplement to *Obesity* in February 2005, which comprised 102 manuscript pages and a total of 603 literature citations.

Specific recommendations are too numerous to list here, but included recommendations for the multidisciplinary care of the weight loss surgical patient, including criteria for surgeon and hospital credentialing, as well as preoperative, intraoperative, and postoperative care recommendations for all aspects of the care of the weight loss surgical patient.

D. Impact of Betsy Lehman I

The recommendations were not only published in a peer-review journal, the findings were abstracted by AHRQ and served as the basis for an international symposium on Patient Safety in Obesity Surgery held in Boston in July 2005. This symposium was subsequently developed into a DVD-based education program and a book. The recommendations have defined the standard of care for weight loss surgery in Massachusetts. Certain programs in Massachusetts have ceased to offer weight loss surgery, whereas others have started up in compliance with the recommendations. Since 2004, accreditation programs have been developed by the American Society of Metabolic and Bariatric Surgery/Surgical Review Corporation and the American College of Surgeons. Many of the criteria for certification by these programs are similar, if not the same as the Lehman Center recommendations. The Centers for Medicare and Medicaid Services made a national coverage decision on weight loss surgery in February 2006 in which they will only cover WLS carried out in facilities that meet accredited standards of excellence developed by these organizations.

E. Betsy Lehman II

Due to a large body of new literature, and identification of new issues that needed to be addressed, the Betsy Lehman Center convened the second Expert Panel on Weight Loss Surgery in 2007. The goal was to update the initial recommendations based on this new literature. The expert panel was increased to 33 members, and the task groups were increased from 9 to 11 (Table 31.2). The Coding and Reimbursement task group was changed to the Policy and Access group to address concerns with regard to policy implications on access to care. Behavioral and Psychological Care was split out as a separate group from the Multidisciplinary Evaluation task group to reflect the importance of this area. An Endoscopic Interventions task group was added to reflect the advent of this new experimental modality. Specific considerations were made for the new US literature of the laparoscopic adjustable gastric band, and the advent of the laparoscopic sleeve gastrectomy as a standalone procedure. A similar methodology to the first panel was followed, and a similar process of expert panel approval was respected. Recommendations will again be published in *Obesity*.

Table 31.2. Task Groups of Betsy Lehman II.

1) Surgical Care
2) Multidisciplinary Evaluation and Treatment
3) Behavioral and Psychological Care
4) Pediatric/Adolescent Weight loss surgery
5) Anesthetic Perioperative Care and Pain Management
6) Nursing Perioperative Care
7) Informed Consent/Patient Education
8) Policy and Access
9) Specialized Facilities and Resources
10) Data Collection
11) Endoscopic Interventions

F. Conclusion

Evidence-based recommendations for best practices in weight loss surgery have been developed by the Betsy Lehman Center Expert Panel on Weight Loss Surgery. These recommendations and similar recommendations based on the available literature and expert opinion have been the cornerstone of the accreditation programs for weight loss surgery. Recommendations and guidelines will need to be continuously updated to reflect new information from the literature, the introduction of new modalities, and additional experience with the care of the morbidly obese patient.

G. Selected References

Lehman Center Weight Loss Surgery Expert Panel. Commonwealth of Massachusetts. Betsy Lehman Center for Patient Safety and Medical Error Reduction. Expert Panel on Weight Loss Surgery: executive report. Obes Res 2005;13:206–226.

Lehman Center Weight Loss Surgery Expert Panel. Commonwealth of Massachusetts. Betsy Lehman Center for Patient Safety and Medical Error Reduction. Expert Panel on Weight Loss Surgery: executive report: Update 2007. Obesity, in press.

32. American Society for Metabolic and Bariatric Surgery (ASMBS) Centers of Excellence Program

Stacy A. Brethauer, Bipan Chand, and Philip R. Schauer

A. Centers of Excellence Concept

In 2003, in response to the public perception of dramatic variability in outcomes after bariatric surgery, the American Society for Metabolic and Bariatric Surgery (ASMBS) established a quality assurance initiative known as the Bariatric Surgery Center of Excellence (BSCOE). Previously, no minimal standards existed for hospitals or surgeons to perform bariatric surgery. ASMBS established an independent, nonprofit organization known as the Surgical Review Corporation (SRC) to establish quality criteria for hospitals and surgeons as well as to evaluate, certify, and monitor individual hospitals and surgeons. The primary goal of the BSCOE is to allow patients, referring physicians, and health insurance carriers to identify hospitals and surgeons that are performing bariatric surgery at a high standard. The secondary goal is to ensure continued quality improvement in all qualifying BSCOE sites. To qualify as a BSCOE, surgeon practices and hospitals are required to submit documentation supporting the fact that they meet facility and practice standards. All sites must pass a rigorous onsite inspection in order to acquire final approval. In addition, all certified BSCOEs must collect and submit selected outcome data periodically for analysis. The following are the specific requirements for obtaining full approval as a BSCOE.

The Bariatric COE program is designed to ensure that:

- Surgery is performed by qualified teams in well-equipped hospitals.
- Each center selects and standardizes its best care.
- Every patient is reported into a uniform database.
- Results be compared and applied to create continuous quality improvement.

The specific goals of the program are to establish:

- Patient safety and advocacy
- A central outcomes database
- A consortium for research
- Improved health plan coverage, lower medical malpractice premiums, and better access to quality care
- The industry gold standard for bariatric surgery excellence

B. Application Process

1. Application is voluntary.
2. For each program that applies, separate applications must be submitted for:

    a. Each individual surgeon
    b. The surgical practice or group
    c. The institution

C. Provisional Status

1. Focuses on the resources of the institution and the training and experience of the surgeon and surgical group.
2. Provisional status is designated for 2 years. Prior to the 2-year deadline, application for full approval is submitted.
3. Requirements for provisional status

    a. Institutional commitment (medical staff and administration) to excellence in the care of bariatric surgical patients documented with regular in-service training and credentialing guidelines.
    b. Expectation that the institution will perform ≥125 bariatric procedures/year.
    c. Expectation that each applicant surgeon will have performed at least 125 bariatric procedures (primary or revisions) lifetime and at least 50 in the preceding 12 months. Applicants may include up to 75 operations performed during their fellowship in this total lifetime count.
    d. The applicant maintains a designated physician medical director for bariatric surgery
    e. The applicant hospital maintains, within 30 minutes of request, a full complement of medical consultants required for the care of the bariatric surgery patient.
    f. The applicant maintains a full line of instruments and equipment required for the care of the bariatric surgical patient including furniture, wheelchairs, operating room tables, beds, radiologic capabilities, surgical instruments, and other facilities suitable for morbidly obese patients.
    g. The applicant institution has a bariatric surgeon who spends a significant portion of his or her efforts in the field of bariatric surgery and who has qualified coverage and support for patient care.
    h. The applicant uses standardized clinical pathways and orders for perioperative care. Each surgeon should have a standardized method for performing bariatric procedures.
    i. The applicant utilizes designated nurse or physician extenders who are dedicated to serving bariatric surgical patients and are involved in continuing education in the care of bariatric patients.

j.   The applicant makes available organized and supervised support groups for all patients who have undergone bariatric surgery at the institution.

k.   The applicant provides documentation of a program dedicated to a goal of long-term patient follow-up of at least 75% for bariatric procedures at 5 years with a monitoring and tracking system for outcomes, and agreement to provide annual outcome summaries to SRC.

4. Designations for provisional status application

a.   Approved. The applicant can apply for full approval within 2 years.

b.   Denied. The applicant can appeal to the Board of Directors. The applicant has 6 months to correct deficiencies.

c.   Monitoring status. This is assigned when case volume appears to be insufficient to meet the minimum institution and surgeon requirements. Applicants are asked to report case volumes in 6 months.

d.   Pending status. Additional information is required to make a decision.

D. Full Approval

1.   Focuses on patient population, procedures performed, and outcomes

2.   Requires a site inspection (tour of facility, interview, chart review, evaluation of the center and quality of care)

3.   Approved for 3 years

4.   Requirements for full approval

a.   Must continue to meet 10 requirements for provisional status

b.   Deficiencies noted during provisional status review are corrected

c.   Changes in the institution or staff since provisional status granted must be reported

d.   Report of academic activities of the surgeons

e.   Surgeons must be board certified

f.   Outcome data for all bariatric surgery patients must be reported in the Bariatric Outcomes Longitudinal Database (BOLD™). BOLD is an internet-based patient outcomes tracking database. It can be used to collect basic outcomes to comply with COE requirements (BOLD-Core™ version) or it can be used as a comprehensive database system to track patients and provide extended data collection (BOLD-Complete™ version)

5. Designations for full approval application

a.   Full approval: Recommendation is forwarded by the Bariatric COE to the ASMBS Executive Council for final consideration and vote

b.   Denied: Placed back on provisional status. Can request application be reviewed again, request a second site visit, or appeal to board of directors

   c.   Pending: Reviewers request additional information or a second site visit

   d.   Probationary status: Fail to meet the requirements after previously receiving designation for full approval. Program has 6 months to rectify the deficiencies to be reinstated

E. Freestanding Outpatient Bariatric Surgery Center of Excellence

1. Surgery center located greater than one mile from tertiary center is considered freestanding.
2. Same provisional status requirements as hospital-based program plus items 3 to 6 below.
3. Low-risk patients only (BMI <55, age <60, weight <425 lbs, no history of deep vein thrombosis or pulmonary embolism, ASA class <4).
4. Outpatient center must perform at least 100 procedures per year.
5. No procedures that include stapling or division of gastrointestinal tract.
6. Must have a written transfer agreement with a tertiary care facility capable of managing bariatric surgical patients.

As of this date, over 250 hospitals and nearly 500 surgeons in the United States have met the standards to become an ASMBS Bariatric Surgery Center of Excellence. Since most of these sites were required to improve their existing program to meet the high standards of the BSCOE program, the quality of care for the bariatric surgery patient throughout the United States has improved as a direct result of this initiative. Aggregate outcome data of more than 55,000 patients collected during qualifying for BSCOE status reveal a hospital mortality of 0.14%, an operative (<30-day) mortality of 0.29%, a readmission rate of 4.75%, and re-operation rate of 2.15%. These perioperative outcomes are quite favorable considering the general high-risk status of many bariatric patients. Continued outcome monitoring will enable further improvement and ultimately result in better care for bariatric surgery patients.

F. Selected References

Champion JK, Pories WJ. Centers of Excellence for Bariatric Surgery. Surg Obes Relat Dis 2005;1(2):148–151.

Pratt GM, McLees B, Pories WJ. The ASBS Bariatric Surgery Centers of Excellence program: a blueprint for quality improvement. Surg Obes Relat Dis 2006;2(5):497–503; discussion 503.

Surgical Review Corporation website at http://www.surgicalreview.org.

33. The American College of Surgeons (ACS) Bariatric Surgery Center Network

Bruce Schirmer

A. Introduction

The American College of Surgeons is the largest organization of surgeons in the United States, and widely held to be the "parent" organization for surgeons in this country. It represents surgeons from all disciplines. The largest component of the membership of the ACS is general surgeons. While general surgeons in the United States have a wide variety of specialty and regional organizations of which they may become members, the ACS remains the single large common organization for the general surgeon in the United States.

Since the ACS holds such a position, its mission includes providing educational and professional services for all its members. The ACS has a Division of Research and Optimal Patient Care. One of the main focal points of that division is programs that help improve the delivery of surgical care in the safest manner possible. In the past, the ACS has, to this end, taken on the role of supervisory organization for quality standards in certain types of facilities that provide surgical services. The first of these organizational roles was for the ACS to develop guidelines for treatment of the critically injured patient. Trauma centers in this country are now classified by a system of levels of care, with designations defined by facilities, staff, and capabilities for caring for the injured patient. Subsequently the ACS took on the role as the organization that provided standards for cancer centers in the United States. Criteria for centers included personnel, facilities, and processes that would improve the delivery of care to the surgical patient with cancer.

The ACS was, through its previous actions in establishing guidelines for and inspections of facilities in trauma and cancer, accepting its role as the single largest organization of surgeons with the capacity to supervise such major programs as well as the professional and social responsibility of providing the highest standards of surgical practice for patients. The Board of Regents of the College began discussions in the fall of 2004 regarding the extension of the "centers" concept to other areas in surgery. It was decided that bariatric surgery would be the first such additional area in the realm of general surgery to which such a system would be developed.

In the fall of 2004, a steering committee for the creation of criteria for centers of excellence for the ACS was established. This ACS Bariatric Surgery Network Planning Committee, headed by Dr. R. Scott Jones, Head of the

Division of Research and Optimal Patient Care of the ACS, began assembling a set of criteria for centers for bariatric surgery. While the committee was in the process of proceeding with determining the final details of the center's system, the Board of Regents officially voted to endorse and move forward with the initiative in February 2005. Criteria for the ACS Bariatric Surgery Centers Network were finalized shortly thereafter. These are outlined in the following.

It is appropriate to mention that the preceding process of establishing centers for bariatric surgery took place while the Surgical Review Corporation, a corporation separate from but closely affiliated with the then American Society for Bariatric Surgery (ASBS), now known as the American Society for Metabolic and Bariatric Surgery (ASMBS), was engaged in a similar process. Having two competing systems was viewed as undesirable by the majority of bariatric surgeons in the United States. Sincere and significant efforts to arrive at a common system agreeable to both parties unfortunately did not meet with success. Currently both systems are functioning to serve the purpose of qualifying bariatric centers in the United States. The potential for a future merger into one common system is felt by the practicing bariatric surgeon to be best arrangement. The ACS is still amenable to reopening such discussions with the potential to resolving differences and achieving this goal.

A recent report published in the *ACS Bulletin* also summarizes the criteria for the ACS Bariatric Surgery Center Network centers, and the reader is referred to it for additional information, including a list of ACS-accredited centers as of August 2007 (33 Level 1, one Level 2, and one outpatient center).

B. Guidelines

The ACS Bariatric Surgery Network Planning Committee relied on several documents and published data to arrive at its criteria for bariatric centers. The Betsy Lehman Center for Patient Safety and Medical Error Reduction had already assembled an expert panel of physicians largely from the state of Massachusetts to create a report on best practices in bariatric surgery. The goal was to establish criteria to maximize safe conduct of bariatric surgery. The report was published in *Obesity Research*. Guidelines for that report were taken from the published literature on bariatric surgery as well as the expertise of the group. In addition to the Betsy Lehman guidelines, a host of other major articles pertaining to patient safety and outcomes regarding bariatric surgery were reviewed by the committee. Available literature that focused on outcomes of bariatric surgery and relationships to factors such as volume, surgeon experience, and others were particularly included for the review by the committee prior to formulating criteria for centers. The Planning Committee was composed not only of bariatric surgeons, but also epidemiologists and experts in outcomes research. Senior bariatric surgeons as well as younger bariatric surgeons recognized for expertise in laparoscopic bariatric surgery were included in the committee. The ACS had two dedicated staff assigned to the project as well. Committee composition is listed in Table 33.1.

Table 33.1. Composition of ACS bariatric surgery network planning committee.

R. Scott Jones, MD, FACS; Head, ACS Division of Research
    and Optimal Patient Care
John Alverdy, MD, FACS
Nancy Birkmeyer, MD, FACS
David Flum, MD, FACS
Matthew Hutter, MD, FACS
Daniel Jones, MD, FACS
Edward Mason, MD, FACS
Ninh Nguyen, MD, FACS
Patrick O'Leary, MD, FACS
Heena Patel, MD, FACS
Bruce Schirmer, MD, FACS
Daniel Smith, MD, FACS
Karen Richards, ACS Staff
Bianca Reyes, ACS Staff

1. Adopting criteria for centers

The first and major concept that the ACS network embraced was that the system would certify centers, but not individual surgeons. The credentialing and privileging of surgeons to practice in any hospital has traditionally been under the jurisdiction of that hospital, and the ACS felt this practice should continue.

The second and equally major concept adopted by the ACS network was that of "levels" for centers. This levels concept was similar to that used for classifying trauma centers by the ACS. A Level 1 center would be a more comprehensive center, whereas a Level 2 center would be one that performed bariatric surgery in an excellent fashion, but in a smaller or less comprehensive setting. A final category for outpatient centers was also designated, in keeping with emerging trends of bariatric practice at the time, and anticipation of them in the future.

The ACS Bariatric Surgery Network Planning Committee adopted various criteria for centers based on available best evidence from the bariatric surgical literature. Considerable debate and discussion surrounded several of the points for center qualification. Once center criteria were finally adopted in the spring of 2005, the ACS Bariatric Surgery Network Planning Committee was converted to the ACS Bariatric Surgery Center Network Advisory Board, composed solely of bariatric surgeons and support personnel from the ACS. Applications for center status were accepted, and the process of reviewing applications was begun.

C. Center Levels and Descriptors

Bariatric Centers in the ACS Network are of three types: Level 1, Level 2, and Outpatient. A subsequent modifier or descriptor of each type of center was later adopted, a new center status. In addition, each center was given a descriptor letter to follow the level number, which described whether or not the center used the National Surgery Quality Improvement Program (NSQIP, see the following for further details) or not. Centers that used this program were labeled "A," whereas those that did not were labeled "B." While the ACS has strongly promoted the use of the NSQIP system for all hospitals, it was felt requiring hospitals to adopt this system, which entails considerable expense to the hospital, might prove excessively burdensome to institutions, which could deter them from participating in the Centers Network system.

1. Level 1 center criteria

Level 1 centers are centers located in large, usually tertiary care hospitals, where patient volume is considerable and bariatric surgery is practiced by at least two bariatric surgeons. A Level 1 center needs to have had a bariatric surgery program in existence for at least 1 and preferably 2 years. A total of no fewer than 125 primary bariatric operations must have been done in the previous 12 months. Such operations must be "standard" bariatric operations, or those recognized by the NIH criteria and insurance payers through the CPT code process as being bariatric surgical procedures. Revisional surgery, involving standard type operations, may also be included. While centers may perform "nonstandard" operations, such operations do not count toward the minimum annual number of operations required, and must not exceed 50% of the volume of bariatric operations at any center.

Level 1 centers must have at least two full-time bariatric surgeons active on the staff of the hospital. The definition of "active" is that the bariatric surgeon performs elective bariatric operations at the hospital and takes call for bariatric surgery cases for the hospital. In order to also qualify as a "bariatric surgeon" in a Level 1 hospital, a surgeon must have performed at least 50 bariatric operations during the previous 12 months. Not all of the procedures need be done at the hospital or medical center for which the bariatric surgeon is counted as a qualified surgeon, for it is recognized that some surgeons work at more than one hospital.

Level 1 centers also must have an environment consistent with the highest level of acute patient care for bariatric surgery. Most often such hospitals are tertiary care hospitals, but this need not be the case if the requirements for care of the bariatric surgery patient are provided at the highest acuity level.

Level 1 centers are expected to be able to treat most if not all qualified bariatric patients, and have the capability of treating the high-risk bariatric patient. Personnel who are required for a Level 1 center include not only those comprising the basic bariatric team (Table 33.2), but also medical and surgical subspecialties that may be required to assist in the optimal care of the high-risk

Table 33.2. Composition of the basic bariatric surgery team.

Bariatric surgeon
Bariatric program coordinator (nurse or physician extender)
Nutritionist
Psychologist
Administrative secretary
Data manager (role may be fulfilled by coordinator)
Primary care physician

and challenging bariatric surgery patient. The constant availability of specially trained or dedicated anesthesiologists on call 24 hours a day, 7 days a week (24/7) is one such personnel requirement. The availability of consulting medical subspecialty services in cardiology, pulmonology, gastroenterology/endoscopy, endocrinology, internal medicine, rheumatology, psychiatry, radiology, gynecology, plastic surgery, thoracic surgery, otorhinolaryngology, orthopedics, and critical care is all expected in a Level 1 center. Level 1 centers are also expected to provide psychologists, bariatric-oriented nurses, nutritionists, and social workers as well as make exercise physiologists available to patients. Usually the nutritionist and psychologist are represented on the core bariatric team as well.

Facilities at Level 1 centers must be of the highest quality for the care of the bariatric surgical patient. The center must provide and maintain a fully staffed and medically equipped intensive care unit capable of treating bariatric surgery patients. The same is true for the operating room, including minimally invasive procedure capabilities. The recovery room must be fully staffed and always available to treat bariatric surgical patients. The endoscopy unit must be staffed and available for use 24/7. The same is true of the emergency room in terms of being able to accommodate bariatric patients. Dialysis capability is necessary. Appropriate imaging equipment for bariatric patients (oversize CT scanners, high weight capacity tilt tables for fluoroscopy, etc.) is required. There must be adequate numbers of inpatient rooms that are specifically built to accommodate bariatric patients, with features such as wide doors, floor-mounted toilets, bed trapezes, oversize bathrooms with wide showers, and specialty bariatric beds. Equipment in the operating room, recovery room, ICU, inpatient unit, and other areas of the hospital as mentioned must include size-appropriate items for the bariatric patient, including oversize gowns, wide blood pressure cuffs, extra long instruments, extra wide chairs and walkers, special transfer devices, and special beds. Seating capacity in hospital common areas, waiting rooms, and offices must be able to accommodate the bariatric patient, as must examining tables and other equipment in both inpatient and outpatient areas of the patient experience.

In addition to equipment and staffing, the staff that serves the bariatric patient population must have sufficient orientation, special training sessions, and other appropriate preparation for dealing with the psychological and physical issues that these patients face during their hospitalization or visit to the facility as an outpatient.

The individuals that comprise the bariatric team are expected to be even more experienced and appropriately trained in the art and science of caring for the bariatric surgical patient. The required number of bariatric surgeons for a Level 1 center is at least two, as mentioned. Surgeons must of course meet the guidelines and qualifications of the local hospital privileging and credentialing committee for practice. Board certification or the equivalent or eligibility is necessary. Documentation of ongoing CME in bariatric surgery is needed for recertification. Case volume must be adequate. Cases done as an assistant may be counted if the assistant plays a role in the perioperative care of the patient (co-manages the patient) as well as participates in the operative procedure. There must be a bariatric program director, who is a bariatric surgeon.

Other key members of the bariatric team include a program coordinator, who is usually a nurse, nurse clinician, or physicians assistant. That person must have adequate medical training and experience in caring for bariatric surgery patients to serve as the major coordinator of care for patients as they go through the process of preoperative preparation, operative procedure, and postoperative care and follow-up. It is also expected that the Level 1 center provide a full time nutritionist for bariatric patients. A psychologist is also an important member of the team, as is a social worker when needed, and of course the patient's primary care physician. The office manager and administrative and/or secretarial support for the program are individuals who must be sensitive to the needs and concerns of the bariatric patient while being attentive to and understanding of the high volume of office calls that this patient population usually produces. A designated and trained individual or individuals from either the physician extender group or the office administrative portion of the team must learn and be responsible for recording careful preoperative, operative, and postoperative data regarding patient outcomes for the ACS bariatric database. There must be ready availability by referral to exercise therapists, plastic surgeons, and medical specialists as listed. Finally, the program must have both the verbal and written pledge of support for its success by the hospital administration, including a documented record of providing appropriate resources when needed.

2. Level 2 center criteria

Level 2 centers differ from Level 1 centers mainly in the size and complexity of the medical facilities and personnel available for the care of the bariatric patient. Level 2 centers must provide appropriate inpatient facilities for all bariatric surgical patients, including the operating room, recovery room, intensive care unit, and intermediate care unit. Outpatient facilities must also be of the same high standards. However, a Level 2 center is not expected to provide 24/7 availability of the entire array of medical specialists. Certain members of the bariatric team may not be full time, such as the nutritionist, but must be available. Facilities appropriate for the community-sized hospital are acceptable as long as they provide for the safe care of the bariatric patient and emergent situations that may arise for those patients. Capability for transfer if a particularly difficult complication arose must be available for patients at a Level 2 center.

3. Patient education and preparation for surgery

While personnel, facilities and equipment are all essential physical and human components of the bariatric program, there must also be a strong process of patient selection, evaluation, preparation, education, and preparation for surgery. Appropriate written educational material must be given to patients well before surgery, and a process of thorough patient education adopted. While no hard and fast rule exists requiring forms of media for materials, many centers use talks, videos, web sites, written tests, and other means to improve and document patient education and knowledge regarding their upcoming bariatric operation.

The process of informed consent prior to bariatric surgery is particularly emphasized as needing to be well documented, especially in terms of informing the patient of the surgeon's experience, the details of the proposed procedure, expected outcomes, and potential common complications and risks. This is true for all levels of centers.

4. Patient selection and preparation

Level 1 centers are expected to be able to provide bariatric surgery services for all patients deemed appropriate candidates for surgery. This includes high-risk patients, male patients, patients with previous abdominal operations, and patients with high BMI and older age. Level 2 centers are not expected to provide services for higher-risk patients, and in fact are only approved for providing services to patients who would not normally be considered high risk. While this latter category has been a challenge to define for the ACS BSCN Committee, current guidelines for appropriate Level 2 center patients are male patients with a BMI less than 50, and female patients with a BMI less than 55. In addition, any patient with a significant history of cardiopulmonary disease, or any major risk factor such as a history of DVT or genetically hypercoagulable state, nonambulatory status, organ failure such as chronic renal failure, or other severe comorbidity that would put the patient in an ASA category 4 status would be grounds for ineligibility at a Level 2 center. Table 33.3 summarizes the major differences between Level 1 and Level 2 centers in terms of facilities, case volume, surgeon number, and patient appropriateness.

The process for selecting patients must be clarified by the center. The surgeon should have the ultimate determination of the decision, but use of a multidiscipline team for patient selection is encouraged. If such a team is not specifically involved in patient selection, they must be used to evaluate patients as indicated preoperatively to determine their appropriateness for bariatric surgery.

5. Quality assurance

All centers, regardless of level, must have a quality assurance program in place. The process and its application to bariatric surgery outcomes must be ·

Table 33.3. Major differences between Level 1 and Level 2 centers.

Category	Level 1	Level 2
Annual case volume	125	25
Number surgeons	2 or more	1
Patients treated	All eligible	Lower risk:
		Males BMI <50
		Females BMI <55
		ASA 3 or less
		No severe cardiopulmonary risks
		No severe other comorbidities
Services	24/7 tertiary care type	24/7 essential services, noncritical services available but not 24/7
Facilities	All tertiary care type	Community hospital type

clarified. Examples of its use are usually asked at the site visit. Protocols for perioperative care of bariatric patients are encouraged, and routine review and modification based on current data and outcomes should be a regular event.

D. Data Collection

Data collection and reporting are requirements for all centers. Whether Level 1 or 2, all bariatric cases must be entered into a database and collected by the ACS. Data belong to the individual center, and comparisons to each center to aggregate data for the entire database are available in order to gauge performance relative to peers. There are currently two systems for collecting bariatric data for either level centers. If a center is already using the National Surgical Quality Improvement Program (NSQIP) program in its hospital, they are a type A center. If the center is not using the NSQIP program, they are a type B center.

The NSQIP involves collection of patient-related data with the ultimate goal of improving patient safety and surgical outcomes through monitoring of results in comparison with others performing similar procedures. The system was initially begun within the Veterans Administration System, and now has been extended to not only tertiary care private hospitals, but hospitals of all varieties and sizes. Patient information includes demographic, preoperative, and postoperative data. Table 33.4 outlines the major components of the data points involved in NSQIP. Trained reviewers record data from an approximately 20% sampling of inpatients. These data are periodically audited for quality assurance. Outcomes for each individual center are risk adjusted based on the mathematical risk adjustment of preoperative coexisting medical problems of the patient population. Thus, a NSQIP center receives their own risk-adjusted outcomes for each of the various operative procedures recorded by the database. Currently general surgery and vascular surgery are so recorded. Bariatric surgery is included in the general surgery reported outcomes for those medical centers in which NSQIP has already been in place.

For ACS Bariatric Surgery Centers, the major difference between type A and B centers is that for the A centers, data already collected for bariatric patients by

Table 33.4. The ACS NSQIP database.

All patients undergoing major surgery
Preoperative data
10 demographic variables
40 clinical variables
12 laboratory variables
Intraoperative data
15 clinical variables
Postoperative data
30-day postoperative mortality
20 categories of 30 day postoperative morbidity
Length of hospital stay

the NSQIP data collectors can be easily transferred into the ACS Bariatric Database. This ACS Bariatric Database is designed to collect patient data, including demographic information, preoperative medical conditions, operative data, and postoperative follow-up data, including morbidity and mortality, resolution of comorbid problems, and weight loss. Each center must submit data on all bariatric patients. Since the NSQIP data system does not necessarily report data on all patients, the bariatric patients not reported by NSQIP would still need reporting by all type A centers. In addition, the NSQIP program collects only 30-day follow-up, and hence any follow-up beyond that, required for all bariatric surgery patients, would need to be reported in the ACS bariatric database.

Each ACS Bariatric Surgery Center must designate at least one data collector who will input data into the ACS bariatric database. In some centers, more than one data collector may be needed if several bariatric surgical groups practice at the center, and have separate office facilities for follow-up visits for patients. The designated reviewer must undergo a training orientation prior to entering data into the database.

While the database questions for the ACS bariatric database were formulated by the ACS Bariatric Surgery Advisory Board as a whole, Dr. Matthew Hutter was the main figure who brought the database to fruition through his efforts in finalizing the data points and working with the database company contracted by the ACS. The database began enrolling patients in September 2007 after training 10 sites as beta test sites. Full rollout for the remainder of the centers is expected in January 2008.

The data obtained through input to the database by centers will, in the future, be the basis for confirming appropriately good outcomes for centers and determining the ability of centers to retain their status as a center. Until now, arbitrary determination of adequate numbers of cases and surgeons has been used as a surrogate for determining center status. Outcomes parameters will also be a more objective means of establishing criteria for becoming a center as well.

1. Patient follow-up

All centers must have a system of patient follow-up that assures adequate safety for the patient and attempts to maximize outcomes of surgical therapy as well. Multiple visits during the first year after surgery are expected, then annual visits at a minimum thereafter. While complete follow-up of all patients is impossible in our current environment, a system that will ensure multiple contacts to the patient who has not returned for scheduled appointments is mandatory. Maximizing follow-up in turn maximizes the quantity and accuracy of follow-up data entered into the database, and reflects with the highest degree of accuracy and certainty the outcomes of bariatric surgical therapy at that center.

E. Special Center Designations

1. Outpatient centers

Recognizing that certain bariatric procedures, particularly laparoscopic adjustable gastric banding at the present time, are often done as outpatient procedures, the ACS designated a special designation for outpatient bariatric surgical centers. These centers must be approved by the same hospital review boards as inpatient hospitals (i.e., JCAHO or equivalent), and have similarly appropriate furniture, equipment, and instruments to accommodate bariatric patients. Surgical equipment and operating rooms must be bariatric capable, as well as minimally invasive capable. If the center does outpatient adjustment of laparoscopic adjustable bands, then the appropriate fluoroscopic radiology equipment to assist with difficult band fills or to determine band tightness must be available, as must personnel to operate them. The required volume of cases for an outpatient center is 100 cases annually. At least one qualified bariatric surgeon must be on the staff. Availability for transfer of patients to an associated inpatient facility should the need arise is necessary. Data reporting and patient follow-up requirements for outpatient centers are similar to those for levels 1 and 2 centers.

2. New centers

Recognizing that there will be growth in the field of bariatric surgery, and that at times an established center could drop from the ranks of the centers if surgeons were to suddenly leave the medical center, the advisory board felt a mechanism needed to be in place for new centers (or old centers that wanted to rejoin the network ranks) to begin performing surgery without an excessively long waiting period in order to qualify. Thus, the category of New Center was defined in 2007. A new center must have the appropriate personnel, equipment, facilities, patient selection, patient education, quality assurance program, and follow-up system as established centers, and must have done at least 25 primary bariatric operations before applying to be a new center. Once a center has applied for this designation, then a site visit is immediately scheduled. Data on outcomes during the first year must be updated and reviewed quarterly, and after one year the center then may achieve either Level 1 or Level 2 status depending on volume and patient selectivity.

F. The Application Process

The process of achieving status as a bariatric center in the ACS Bariatric Surgery Center Network involves preparation and fulfilling the criteria for approval of one of the levels of centers. If a medical center feels they have achieved such preparation and have met the criteria for center status, then an application is filed with the ACS office requesting provisional approval as a center. The initial application asks for basic information on the center, whether or not the hospital is an approved (i.e., JCAHO or comparable) hospital, bed capacity, ICU capacity, occupancy rate, and the capacity of those beds for housing bariatric patients. A letter of support for the bariatric surgery program by the administration must accompany the application. The center is asked to list bariatric surgeons and their case volumes for the previous 2 years. Similarly, the volume of bariatric surgical procedures done in each of the 2 previous years at the center is requested. Checklists for the availability of supporting medical services must be completed, and their availability. Specific questions on bariatric patient selection and education, follow-up, and the hospital's current use or not of the NSQIP system as well as any currently used databases for bariatric surgery outcomes are asked. Outcomes data in terms of mortality, morbidity, and readmission rates must be supplied in the application as well.

An application fee of $10,000 must accompany the completed application. Once this is done, the application is sent to a subgroup of the ACS consisting of four members. These reviewers vote to approve, approve with conditions or pending correction of issues, or disapprove of the application. Once the application has achieved approval, a site visit is scheduled. With the ACS BSCN system, all site reviews are performed by a trained bariatric surgeon. Site reviewers are bariatric surgeons of known reputation who have volunteered to serve in this role. Prior to performing any reviews, they undergo a full-day training session at ACS headquarters. Reviewers are selected to minimize likelihood of conflict of interest in terms of geographic proximity to the site, but also the distance from the site visitors residence to the site visited is attempted to be kept to a minimum. Any concerns regarding objectivity or conflict of interest by the site reviewer that are raised by the site to be visited result in an alternate reviewer being selected. The site and/site visitor arrange a mutually convenient date for the visit.

The actual site visit requires several hours, usually the better part of a working day. The site visitor has an initial interview with the entire group of individuals providing bariatric surgical services, including surgeons, administrators, program coordinators, nutritionists, and others involved in the program. Overall aspects of the program are discussed, including patient selection process, overall progress of the patient from initial visit to surgery, personnel involved in the bariatric team, operations offered, follow-up plan and data collection, and improvement process. The reviewer often may have specific questions regarding the site based on the initial application that was filed. Once this session is completed, the reviewer then tours and inspects the various areas of the hospital, including the operating rooms, recovery rooms, ICU, endoscopy unit, emergency room, inpatient unit, radiology suite, dialysis unit, and outpatient clinic areas. Interviews with personnel in those areas are conducted to determine the usual approach to handling the bariatric patient. Facilities are inspected with specific interest toward their capability of accommodating the bariatric patient. The site reviewer then reviews a number of medical records of bariatric surgery patients, including any deaths or major complications that have occurred during the past year. A final session with the very key individuals involved in the program usually concludes the visit.

The site reviewer then files a report of the site visit to the ACS office. The site visit report is circulated to a group of advisory board members. These members then review the findings and recommendations and vote to either accredit, accredit with reservations, accredit pending correction of certain issues, or not accredit. The majority vote determines the decision.

G. Center Obligations

Once a center has been accredited as a member of the ACS Bariatric Surgery Center Network, it must fulfill its obligations to adhere to the principles of patient care which it had been doing at the time of the site visit, or improve deficiencies cited. Data on all bariatric surgery patients must be reported to the ACS bariatric database. A designated data entry person for each approved site must be identified and trained by the ACS before data entry may begin. For most centers, this process is currently just being initiated as the ACS bariatric database has only recently become available for data entry. If the site is an NSQIP center, then the data collected by NSQIP data collectors relative to bariatric patients may be automatically transferred into the ACS bariatric database.

Outcomes data from all centers will be reviewed on a semiannual basis for all centers by the ACS bariatric database oversight group. This group will report significant deviations from expected norms for any center. Centers that are so identified will be notified and given the opportunity to improve their outcomes over the next 6-month period. Failure to do so will result in suspension or potential dismissal of the center from the network, depending on the severity of the deviation. Similarly, at this time, until more outcomes are available, a center whose volume or number of surgeon status falls below the required level for a Level 1 center could be recategorized as a Level 2 center. The ACS BSCN advisory committee has set a goal to eventually eliminate volume as a surrogate for quality, but the extent to which quality outcomes must be maintained before volume is dismissed has yet to be determined.

H. Summary

The ACS Bariatric Surgery Center Network has been established. Criteria for center acceptance have been established and the process for admitting and certifying centers has proved successful. The function and role of the advisory committee has been determined. These processes have proved to be dynamic ones, with some changes in the initial guidelines being made as the process evolved and role and function of the committee and the system evolving as the system transitions to including data reporting as the main focus of quality. Throughout the process, however, the ACS system has espoused and promoted the goals of the Network as being improvement in the care of the bariatric surgery patient.

I. Selected References

Fink AS, Campbell DA Jr, Mentzer RM Jr, et al. The National Surgical Quality Improvement Program in non-veterans administration hospitals: initial demonstration of feasibility. Ann Surg 2002;236:344–353.

Kelly J, Tarnoff M, Shikora S, et al. Best care recommendations for surgical care in weight loss surgery. Obes Res 2005;13:227–233.

Khuri SF, Daley J, Henderson WG. The comparative assessment and improvement of quality of surgical care in the Department of Veterans Affairs. Arch Surg 2002;137:20–27.

Khuri SF, Daley J, Henderson W, et al. The Department of Veterans Affairs' NSQIP: the first national, validated, outcome-based, risk-adjusted, and peer-controlled program

for the measurement and enhancement of the quality of surgical care. National VA
Surgical Quality Improvement Program. Ann Surg 1998;491–507.

Schirmer B, Jones DB. The American College of Surgeons Bariatric Surgery Center
Network: establishing standards. Bull Amer Coll Surg 2007;92(8):21–27.

Index